REFLEXOLOGY
THE THEORY AND PRACTICE

Ann Gillanders

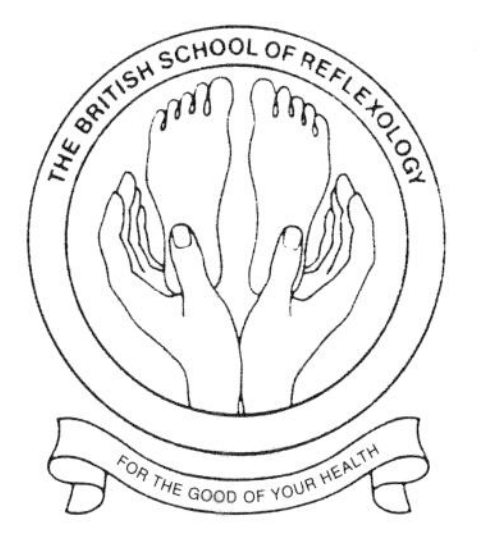

First published 1994
Reprinted 1995, 1997

ISBN 0 9511868 2 5

Prepared for publication by
Jenny Lee Publishing Services, Bishop's Stortford, Herts.
Design and artwork by Gillian Glen.
Illustrations by Eleanor Tanner.
Cover design by Jonathan Barnard.
Typeset by AlphaSet, Hatfield Broad Oak, Hertfordshire.
Printed and bound in Great Britain by The Alden Press, Oxford.

For details of professional courses in reflexology, contact:

The British School of Reflexology
The Holistic Healing Centre
92 Sheering Road
Old Harlow
Essex CM17 0JW

Telephone number: (01279) 429060

Contents

About the author

ANN GILLANDERS is the Principal of the British School of Reflexology. She and her brother Tony Porter were the true pioneers of Reflexology some twenty years ago, and were responsible for the development of Reflexology throughout the United Kingdom.

Ann's career has been both extensive and varied, although directed entirely to the fields of medicine and creativity.

In 1973 she was introduced to Reflexology. At that time it was a completely unknown science, and often ridiculed. Ann trained with Dwight Byers, Director of the International Institute of Reflexology, qualified, and established a large practice in Harlow, where she still practises today.

In 1979 she undertook a teacher-training course with Dwight Byers. She then became Director of the International Institute of Reflexology, where she promoted Reflexology and set up the United Kingdom side of that Institute, establishing training schools in London, Manchester, Switzerland, Paris and Israel.

In 1986 she founded the British School of Reflexology, which has established schools in London, Harlow, Nottingham, Bristol, Harrogate, Scotland and Geneva.

In 1989 she studied Acupressure and Remedial Massage with Dr Louie Chung, Director of the School of Oriental Medicine, and obtained a Diploma.

She has written *Reflexology, The Ancient Answer to Modern Ailments*, *No Mean Feat* and, most recently, this technical training manual, *Reflexology, The Theory and Practice*.

Introduction

Foot reflexology has now been proved to be a very safe and effective way of helping the body to heal itself, and we are able to treat most of the everyday problems which a patient would consult his or her GP about with tremendous results.

Touch therapies are growing in popularity, and the one-to-one communication which reflexology offers has tremendous advantages in stimulating the healing process. For whatever reasons, we do know that patients treated with foot reflexology feel better and enjoy a new-found mental and physical relaxation. Biological and psychological disorders often leave them after they seek the help of a reflexologist.

I have been involved now for some 20 years in the treatment of patients, the training of therapists throughout the world, writing books and unfolding the mysteries attached to the success of reflexology. I am sure that in years to come it will be shown that reflexology stimulates an energy flow in the body and an improvement of nerve and blood supply, and a great relaxation invades the body. As we all know, tension is at the seat of disease. Medical doctors today are accepting more and more that the stresses of modern living are responsible for the disorders of the body.

There are over 7,000 nerve endings in each foot. Maybe this fact, more than any other, explains why we feel so much better when our feet are treated and so miserable when our feet are in an uncomfortable state. Corns and calluses have an adverse effect on the body, and I am sure we have all experienced a situation when we have walked for too long around a busy town on a hot summer's day in new shoes; at the end of that day, we feel ill all over. I have heard it said that 'the pains in her feet were reflected in her face'.

The purpose of writing this technical training manual is to produce a 'Bible' for the practitioner and a training manual for the student, and to impart to those who have a vested interest in reflexology the vast amount of knowledge and experience that I have attained in my long years involved full-time in the development of reflexology.

I still get a tremendous thrill from seeing the benefits that reflexology can achieve in the most chronic situations and the excitement stimulated by our well-trained practitioners, who go out into the world, develop large practices and further the benefits of reflexology even more.

Good health is a gift, and I am sure that eventually the day will come when reflexology will not only be used for treating illness but will also be employed by the public as a way of maintaining good health.

Dorsal

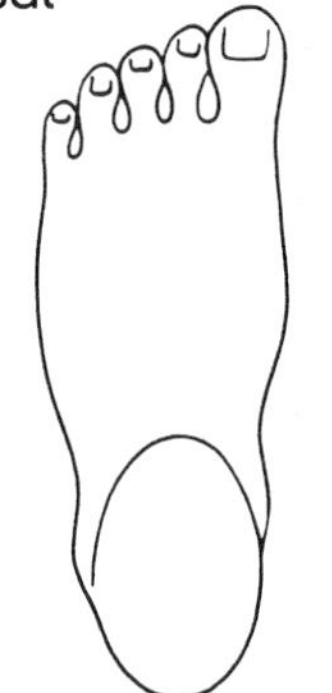

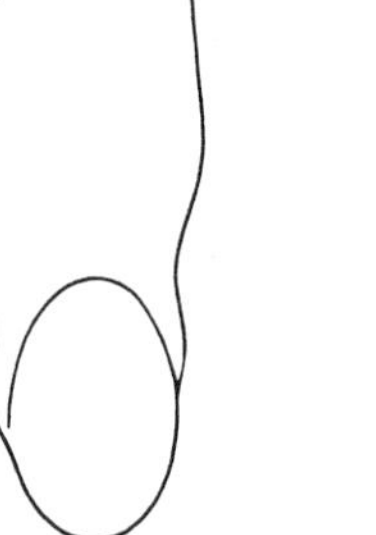

Plantar

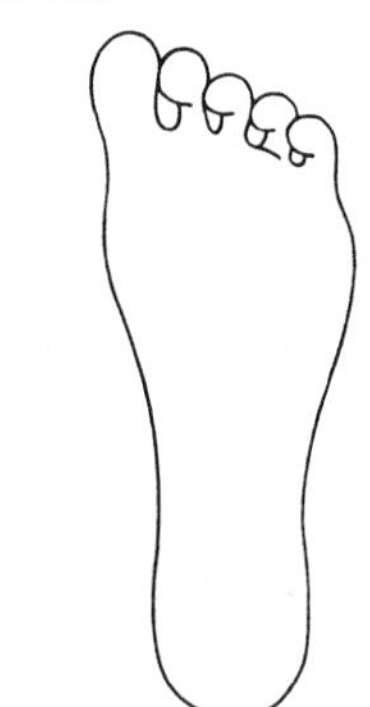

Medial

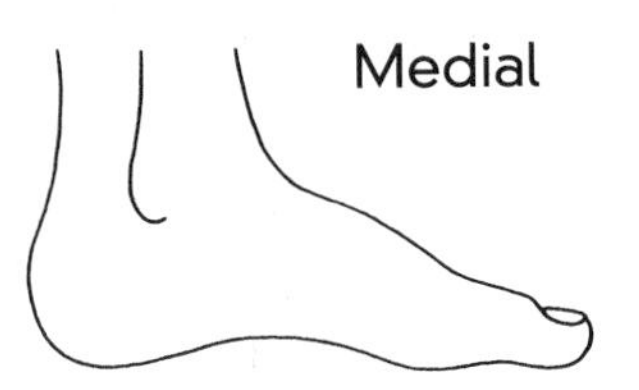

Lateral

Multiple views of the feet

The organisation of this book

Chapters 4 to 13 describe the systems of the body. Each of these chapters begins with a full description of the relevant system. This is followed by a section on practical procedures. Finally there are case studies to show how reflexology has helped someone with a problem in the particular system of the body. Before reading the section on practical procedures study the notes below, which apply to all the practical procedures.

Remember: when there is a duplicated area which is identical in both feet only outline drawings relating to one foot will be shown.

It is essential to adopt the following professional procedures when working on the feet.

Right foot

- When starting to work on the right foot you must support the foot in your left hand and work from the medial to the lateral sides of the foot with the right thumb.
- As you change direction, you must support the right foot with your right hand and, using the left thumb, work back from lateral to medial.

Left foot

- When starting to work on the left foot you must support the foot in your right hand and use the left thumb as you work from the medial to the lateral sides of the foot.
- As you change direction you must support the left foot with the right hand and work back from the lateral to medial with the right thumb.

- Support the top of the foot when working above the waistline.
- Support the heel of the foot when working areas below the waistline.
- To work the medial side of the foot hold the foot in an outward direction supporting the lateral side of the foot.
- When working the lateral side of the foot hold the foot in an upward direction supporting the medial side.
- It is absolutely essential to maintain the habit of working all areas in both directions, exactly as indicated in the following chapters which give you detailed practical instruction on how to work out and identify the way the feet exactly mirror the human body.
- *By covering all areas completely there is no possibility of any reflex areas being 'missed'. Reflex points are the size of pinheads!*

CHAPTER 1 Zones

Zones are longitudinal lines of energy ascending from the feet to the brain. Reflexology is based on zone therapy. As we apply pressure to the feet, we are working on this basis, stimulating these lines which have a rejuvenating and healing effect on the whole of the human body.

We have ten zones, five on each foot, representing a simple numbering system, with the big toe as zone one, the second zone two, the third zone three, the fourth zone four and the fifth zone five. The fingers link up to the zones in the same way, with the thumb being zone one and the little finger zone five (see Figure 1.1).

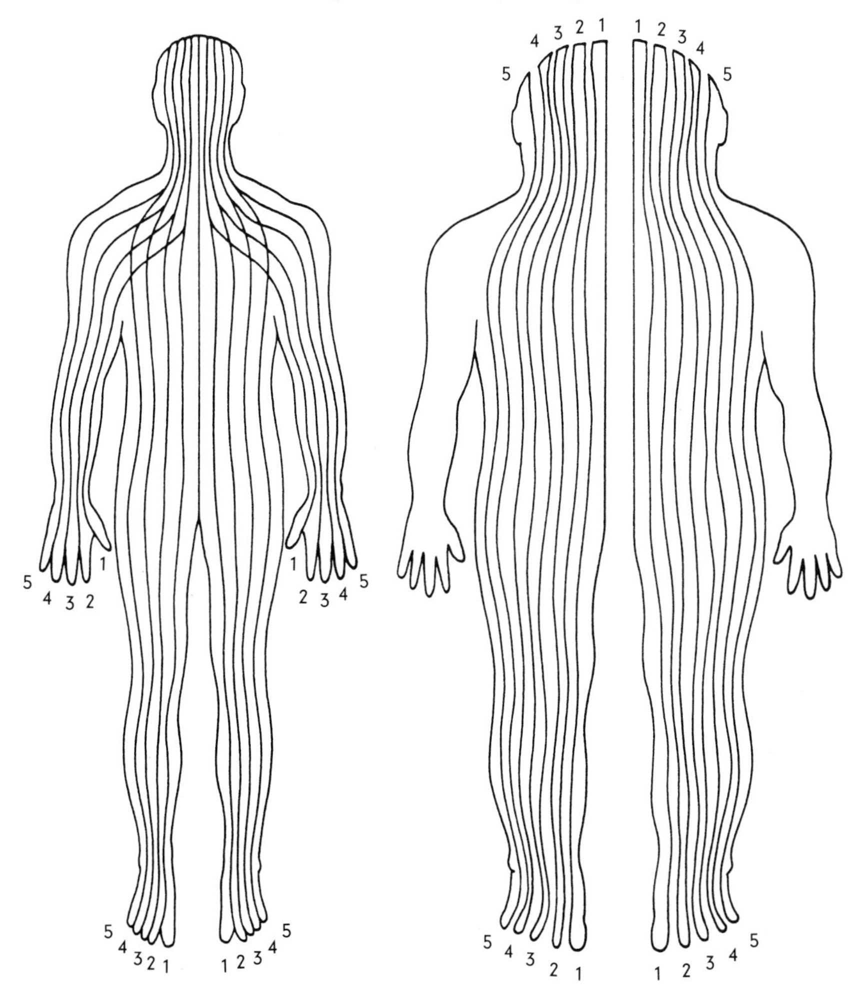

Figure 1.1 There are ten zones in the body running from the toes to the brain, five on either side of the spine. The zones form a simple numbering system with zone one represented by the big toe and thumb, and zone five by the fifth toe and fifth finger.

Zones are distributed through the body like slices. As we work on the plantar side of the feet, we are automatically working through the whole of the human body. A sensitivity in any one spot of the foot creates an imbalance in the entire length of that zone.

Zone one is the most powerful zone in the body because within that zone are many vital functions and parts of the human body. Firstly, we have the all-important central nervous system, spine and brain. The pituitary gland, which is said to be the first gland formed at conception, is the 'master of the orchestra' and is responsible for all the glandular secretions. Our nose is in zone one and obviously, without that important aperture, we would not have the ability to breathe. The mouth is equally important. In zone one we have the commencement of the solar plexus, which is a nerve complexity that lies just behind the stomach and is said to be formed very early after conception. Our reproductive organs are in zone one, and are essential, obviously, for life itself.

You will therefore find, when working on people's feet, that the first zone is always the most sensitive. Many sensitivities in this area are caused by back conditions, but, as has been explained in the previous paragraph, there is immense sensitivity contained in this zone.

The principle of reflexology is to find and work out the sensitive spots in the feet by an alternating pressure of thumb and sometimes the index finger on all parts of the foot.

Refinement of the pressure and consistent control is of great importance in achieving a result. All too frequently I hear of people having received a treatment and getting absolutely no results whatsoever. When treated by a properly qualified practitioner, they are then quite amazed at the outstanding and quick improvement they get in their health problem.

The guidelines of the feet

Apart from the study of zones, we need to understand the guidelines of the feet and their relativity to the parts of the body. In order to practise reflexology, it is essential to have an accurate understanding of these guidelines, which are quite easily identified by certain outstanding features in the feet, and are shown in Figure 1.2.

The **diaphragm line** is found under the bases of the metatarsals. A distinguishing feature is that the colour of the skin on the metatarsal area is quite remarkably different from the underside of the instep. The darker skin is above our diaphragm area and the lighter skin below, so there is almost an identifying line, as if nature intended to help.

The **waist line** is found by running your finger along the lateral side of the foot and feeling a small, bony protrusion about midway. When we find this protrusion we then draw a line across the foot; this area is normally in the narrowest part of the foot.

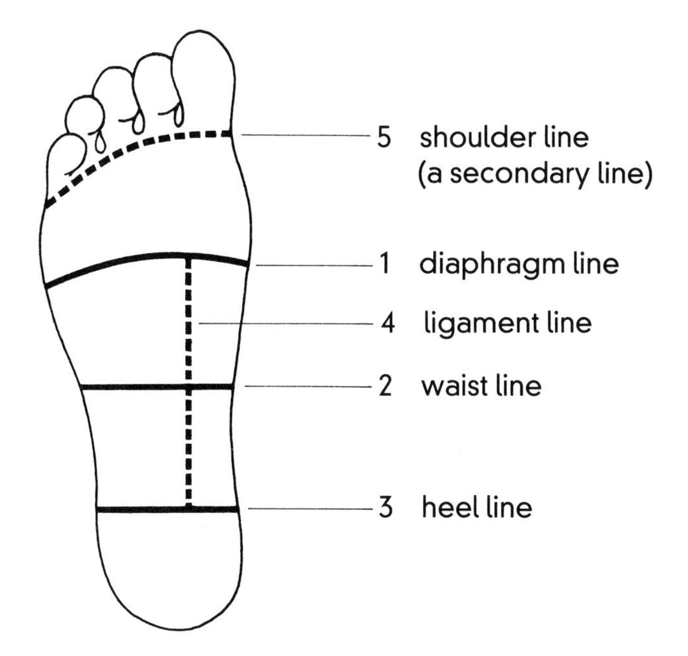

Figure 1.2 Guidelines in the feet

The **heel** or **pelvic line** is found by drawing an imaginary line from the ankle bones on either side of the foot and crossing over the base of the heel, as shown in Figure 1.2.

The **ligament line** is the ascending line which is on the plantar ligament, that taut, elastic-like structure that you can feel if you retract your big toe. Upon this tendon we draw our ligament line.

The **secondary line** is found just below the bases of the toes, and we refer to this as the **shoulder line**.

Reflex responses

A reflex is an involuntary response to stimulus; more particularly, it is a reflex action of an organ, muscle or gland. Reflexes are specific, predictable and purposeful. The reflex response of an organ can take place only if the neural pathway between the point of stimulation and the corresponding organ is intact, with no blockage, or if the pathway can be cleared forcibly by a passing impulse.

Then there is the reflex arch. This neural pathway passes through neurones which are actually the nerve cell (the structure and functional unit of the nervous system). Its main function is to conduct impulses initiated by stimuli. By pressing certain points on the feet we are starting afferent impulses. The term 'afferent' means 'to bear' or 'conduct inwards towards the centre'. Messages are given to the nerve cells, and they in turn transmit into the body to the central stations.

What is a stimulus?

It is any agent or factor able to evoke responses in the organism, even inducing a physiological change. In our work stimulus means contact and pressure which initiates an impulse of a message transmitted through nerve fibres. Thus pressure applied to the nerve ending constitutes a stimulus. The stimulus sets in motion a nerve impulse, an electro-chemical impulse which effects a change in nervous processes. Nerve impulses travel at the rate of about 270 miles per hour, whilst electricity travels at the speed of light.

Our bodies are an electro-chemical plant which is in motion throughout the day and night. We know that all living activities of the human system depend on protoplasm, and that contraction and relaxation are essential to vitality and to life itself. The blood vessels too must be resilient and able to contract and relax automatically if they are to remain functional.

Obstructions in the energy lines

Reflexology teaches that every organ and every gland depends for its survival upon this ability to contract and relax. When an obstacle is placed in the energy channel, as when acid crystals, wastes or unused calcium deposits form on the delicate nerve endings of the feet, the energy flow is impeded and the organ it serves is then adversely affected.

Obstructions in the energy lines and fields register pain, and in certain conditions create limitations in motion and functions; for example, a stiff neck or a painful back. Energy blockage also interferes with blood circulation and this is usually first noticed in the extremities. Hands may become stiff, cold and often painful. Waste products accumulate at the lowest point of gravity, which can be distinctly felt under the thumb and fingers as you work on the feet. There is no substitute for the human hand. No machine can give you this information, and that is why I am totally against all forms of electrical stimulating machines and devices to assist in the treatment of reflexology. We have far too many machines in our modern, everyday twentieth-century life, so it is vital that we now reach back to the natural ways of healing. Hands were in fact meant for healing.

Reflexology as a form of treatment is very rapid in its results. Many a patient can come into the surgery hardly able to walk as a result of a back condition and find that, after the treatment, they are already freed from pain and disability. Generally speaking, chronic conditions require longer treatment time, and the more acute conditions respond quite dramatically and need less frequent treatment.

CHAPTER 2 Your feet – the mirror of your body

The feet are really nothing less than the mirror of the body. The feet are miraculous structural masterpieces, exquisitely and beautifully designed, perfectly co-ordinating many components. Among these are muscles, tissue, 26 bones, 100 ligaments, 20 muscles and an intricate network of nerves and blood vessels. These marvellous structures also reflect totally our state of health. The condition of our feet and the way we use them reveals our physical and mental state and influences not only their own performance but the functioning of our mind and body as well. How we think and act has a direct bearing on how our feet do their job. Likewise, how we treat our feet influences our mental and physical health. It is a two-way street, a reciprocal relationship.

Foot problems

Abuse of the feet and the consequent foot misalignments, which cause blisters, bunions, calluses and corns, often cause, in turn, general fatigue and bodily aches. Conversely, systemic or general body disorders, such as rheumatoid arthritis, diabetes, multiple sclerosis and some types of heart disease, show up first in the feet, causing them to hurt some time before the malfunctioning organs have exhibited other symptoms. Foot pain can indeed camouflage serious diseases, so foot discomfort of any kind demands immediate attention, not only to the foot but to the rest of the body. What may appear to be merely a foot problem could in fact be a symptom of a systemic disease. Medical statistics reveal that two out of three people are plagued with one or more foot problems, so let's look at some of them.

Athlete's foot

Although not a disease in itself, athletes foot represents an entire set of symptoms – scaling between the toes, an itching sensation and a softening of the flesh are the most common of them. It may initially be the result of a fungus, but, if it becomes chronic, roughening of the skin can follow. Known technically as hyperkeratomycosis, which is a thickening and hardening of the external layer of the skin, athlete's foot occurs more frequently in men than women; it may be a local problem; it can also be the result of an allergy, a drug overdose or sunburn. Naturopathic doctors believe that athlete's foot is exacerbated by the body's poor elimination of waste; that is, the skin, lungs, bowel and kidney are not doing their eliminating job very efficiently. Therefore the feet are used as an area of elimination and, through the perspiration, which is normally heavily made up of a very highly proteinous material, the virus which creates athlete's foot thrives in abundance. Often, attention to the body's eliminating processes, in the form of fast extra exercise, hot and cold showers, and body scrubs, gives the body a chance to eliminate its waste through the proper channels, and allows the athlete's foot to disappear.

Bunions

Bunions are another foot problem, the predisposition to which might be inherited, but we do know too that a bunion can develop from poorly fitted shoes. In some, but not in all cases, the 'bursa' or sack over the joint of the big toe becomes inflamed and swollen, sometimes twisting the big toe under the two next to it. When working on a person with such a condition and for whom it is painful, you must work on the corresponding place on the hand. Pressure must not be applied to painful, swollen areas.

Corns and calluses

It is estimated that millions of people suffer from corns and calluses. They can be the result of friction, abnormal foot structure, systemic problems, or even arise through imbalance of mental or emotional upsets. A chiropodist or podiatrist will usually prescribe salicylic acid plasters to remove corns and calluses. Caster oil rubbed twice daily into the affected area softens the corn or callus so that it can eventually be peeled off with the fingers. Other home remedies one might use are the application of a thin slice of lemon fastened with a sticking plaster or adhesive tape and left for the night, or one could apply a piece of cotton dipped in witch hazel to the area for the night. After a number of applications over a period of days the skin usually softens enough to remove the corns and calluses gradually.

Verrucæ

A friend of mine who is a very good chiropodist informs me that a good first-aid remedy for the removal of verrucae is to cut a small square from the skin of a banana, place the inside of the skin onto the area where the verruca is situated and cover it with a piece of sticking plaster. Repeat and replace with a fresh piece daily, and within a week the verruca evidently falls out. I certainly think this would be worth trying if you or somebody in your family is suffering from a verruca.

Fallen arches

Many people are born with a predisposition to fallen arches but may never suffer from them. Arch supports may be helpful in certain circumstances, but specifically designed exercises are preferable. It is interesting to note that through the centuries superstitions or myths have developed about the arches of the feet. One such myth is that high arches are a sign of aristocratic descent. Low arches may be an ethnic characteristic and yet cause no pain. Most people of African origin have flat feet but almost never have the foot pain associated with them. Millions of people have exceptionally low or flat arches but have had no pain or foot problems. The condition is not necessarily abnormal, and whether one's arches are high or low is not of primary importance. It is true that strong arches are important for healthy feet and posture, but flat feet are not always a problem.

Rheumatoid arthritis

In its early stage rheumatoid arthritis may appear as pain, stiffness or swelling of the joints of the feet. Tiny lumps beneath the skin known as subcutaneous nodules may appear as early warning signs of this serious ailment. You can feel these nodules very distinctly under your thumb or fingers. Press gently, because it may cause discomfort if pressure is exerted too enthusiastically, particularly during the first treatment session. When the disease has reached the degenerative, chronic stage, deformities such as hammer toes and bone spurs may appear.

Gout

Appearing more frequently in men than in women, gout is one of the common forms of arthritis. It is possible to be genetically predisposed to arthritic ailments. Even though people who are so disposed have a so-called 'arthritic factor' in their blood, it does not mean that the disease has to develop. Its appearance is often marked by a sudden change in the big toe which becomes shiny, swollen, inflamed and extremely painful. This initial point of irritation is usually the junction of the metatarsal and the phalangeal joint, but other joints in the feet may also be affected. While at first, perhaps mistakenly, it is viewed as a local problem, eventually gout comes to be known for what it is. Gout is caused by a disturbance in the uric acid metabolism which results in the build-up of water in the body. Because of the excess of waste products in the system, insoluble uric acid salts accumulate in the blood around the joints and in the tissues in the form of crystalline deposits which one can feel when they are pressed. Medical authorities indicate that merely being 10 per cent overweight is enough to trigger a pre-existing asymptomatic condition. Thus individuals who watch their weight and get adequate exercise are less likely to develop gout.

Cardiovascular diseases

These affect the heart and circulatory system and may cause pain, swelling and a burning sensation in the feet if the blood circulation is impaired.

Arteriosclerosis

This is the hardening and thickening of the arteries, which seriously reduces blood flow, with the consequent loss of oxygen to the tissues of the feet and removal of deoxygenated blood. This leads to poor gaseous interchange in the tissues. Difficulty in walking, pain when the feet are at rest, ulcers and infections, loss of hair on the legs and thickening of the nails, particularly on the big toes, are all clues to the presence of this disorder.

Other disorders

Swelling and oedema in the feet and legs can be caused by *heart inadequacy*. Body fluids then accumulate in the extremities since they are restricted in their flow. An early symptom of *diabetes* is often a numbness and tingling sensation in the feet. *Ulcers* may develop on the soles, and if infections occur they heal very slowly. Symptoms of *neurological problems* or nerve disorders, even *brain lesions* can appear in the feet in the form of lack of co-ordination, and muscle weakness.

Care of the feet

If you give your feet the kind of care they deserve, the entire system will benefit from mental ease, and general good health will be easier to achieve. Here are some tips on the proper care of the feet.

- Insist on wearing shoes about half an inch (1.3cm) longer than your foot.
- Buy shoes in the afternoon; one's feet expand during the day, particularly in hot weather.
- Leather shoes or fitted sandals are best.
- If you wear socks they should be wool or cotton and, again, half an inch (1.3 cm) longer than your feet.
- After bathing, dry the feet carefully between the toes and use some form of massage oil.
- Cider vinegar is an excellent antiseptic preparation for the feet. All you need is about two tablespoons of cider vinegar in a litre of warm water in which to soak your feet and it will have excellent remedial benefits.
- Do not wear tight-fitting bands at the top of stockings as these restrict your circulation.
- Walking is the best form of exercise.

Two important jobs the feet perform are supporting and maintaining one's posture and propelling the body into whichever direction one desires. The big toe is responsible for helping to control balance, along with the intrinsic muscles of the foot. It is estimated that the force to which each foot is subjected during a single day is equivalent to approximately 600 tons for a 150-pound (68 kilo) person. Did you also realise that within a lifetime the average person walks to the moon and back?

The approach I have taken in writing this book is a totally holistic one: I have written on reflexology, its comparisons to orthodox and complementary medicines, how the body performs in sickness and in health, and I hope I have provided a very good understanding of disease. It is not possible to become a practitioner and learn solely the use of the practical side of reflexology without a deep insight into the theoretical values of medicine, anatomy and physiology, and a true understanding of the meaning of disease and good health.

Everyone who experiences reflexology can benefit from it, but not all will recover completely. No matter what may be done in terms of pressure therapy, some people will continue to eat the wrong food, drink the wrong beverages, refuse to give up smoking, drinking, or taking drugs. These people refuse to alter their mental attitudes about themselves and the world, and so they cannot be helped. We apply specific techniques to induce relaxation, restore proper circulation nerve supply and, most important of all, to restore nature's balance.

CHAPTER 3 Relaxation exercises and thumb technique

Relaxation exercises

Relaxation exercises are special techniques used at the beginning of a treatment, during a treatment and to end a treatment session. They are used to enhance relaxation, and to give the foot maximum movement, and can be used if a specific system in the body creates extra sensitivities in the feet, which may cause a little discomfort to the patient. If we follow the pressure technique with a relaxation exercise, this is very soothing to the patient.

The relaxation exercises are also very useful to students in training, as it gets them used to handling feet and to maintaining contact with the patient throughout the treatment.

Side-to-side relaxation Supporting the foot at the top, use a rocking, side-to-side movement (see Figure 3.1).

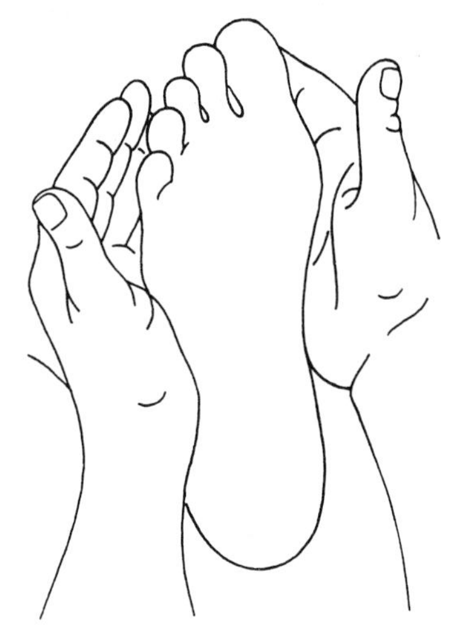

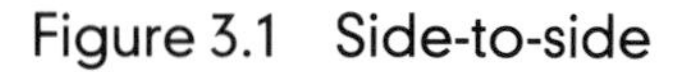

Figure 3.1 Side-to-side

Diaphragm relaxation When beginning with the right foot, place the right thumb on the commencement of the diaphragm line. As you move the thumb outwards towards the lateral side of the foot, bend the toes downwards onto your thumb. At no time should the thumb leave the surface of the foot. This is a great relaxant to the diaphragm muscle, and produces a nice, slow, rhythmic breathing. Change direction and place the left thumb on the lateral edge of the diaphragm line and work back to the medial side (see Figure 3.2).

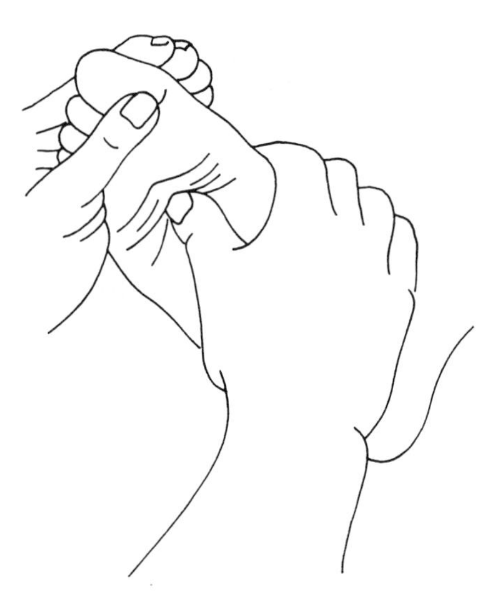

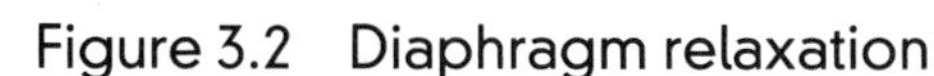

Figure 3.2 Diaphragm relaxation

Metatarsal kneading Commence on the right foot, place the right fist on the right foot, place the left hand over the front of the foot, using a pushing movement from the plantar side, and a gentle squeezing movement from the dorsal side; this is a combined movement – both must be in harmony with each other (see Figure 3.3).

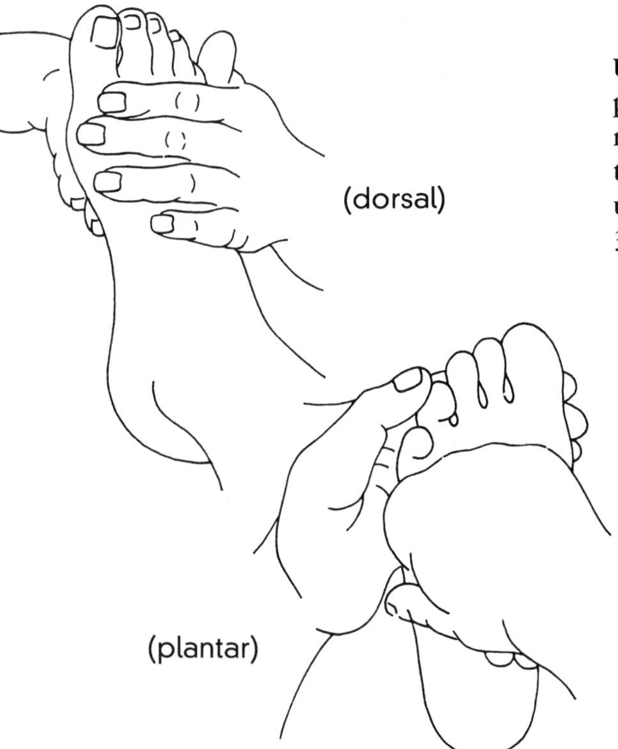

Figure 3.3 Metatarsal kneading

Ankle freeing Commence with the right foot, use both hands and rock the foot with a side-to-side motion. This is excellent for loosening up stiff ankles (see Figure 3.4).

Figure 3.4 Ankle freeing

Undergrip Begin with the right foot and place the left hand under the ankle (the thumb must be on the lateral side of the foot). Turn the foot in an inward direction, being sure to use a light circling movement (see Figure 3.5).

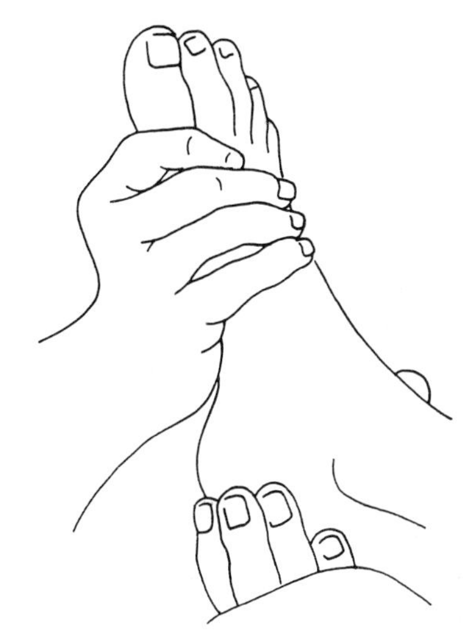

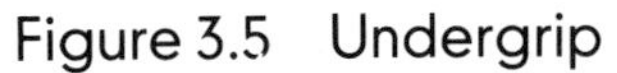

Figure 3.5 Undergrip

Overgrip Using exactly the same technique as before, place the left hand over the top of the ankle, again making sure that the thumb of the left hand is on the outside edge of the foot. This is a very useful technique to use for swollen ankles (see Figure 3.6).

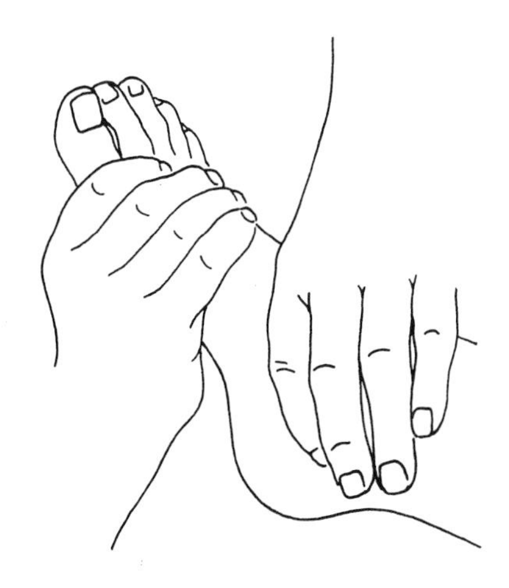

Figure 3.6 Overgrip

Foot moulding Support the right foot (this time from the lateral edge of the foot). Sandwich the foot between your two hands and gently rotate both hands. The motion is identical to the movement of the wheels of a train (see Figure 3.7).

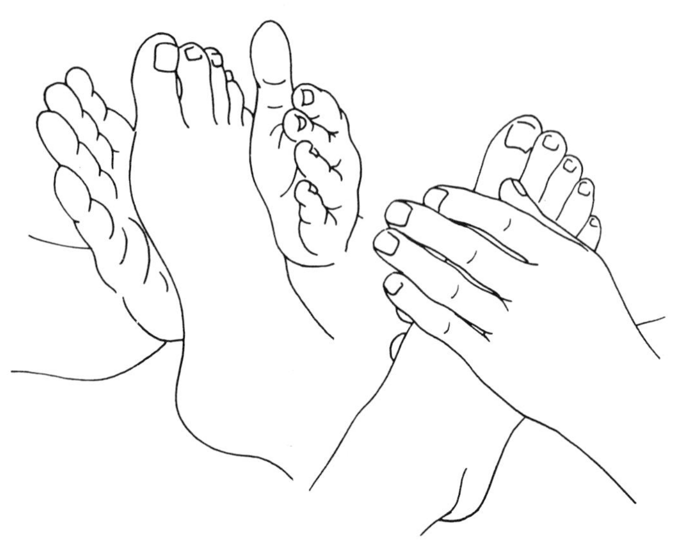

Figure 3.7 Foot moulding

Rib cage Pressing in with the two thumbs on the right foot, use all the fingers of both hands and creep around the dorsal side of the foot (see Figure 3.8).

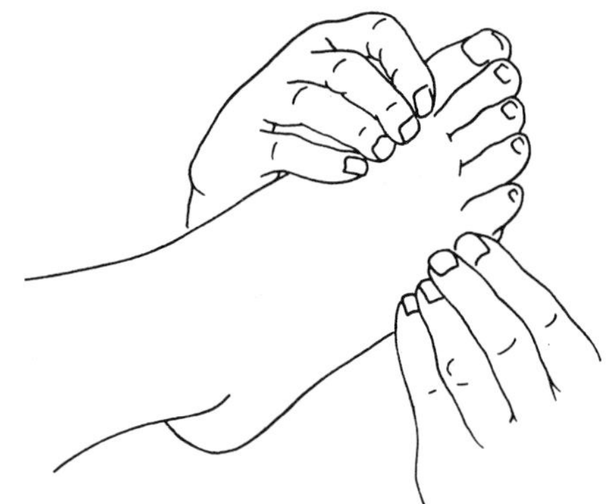

Figure 3.8 Rib cage

The thumb technique

The movement that we need to acquire with our thumb, in particular, is a forward creeping movement, bending from the first joint of the thumb (see Figure 3.9).

- We do *not* rotate in circles, hold a deep pressure for any length of time to any reflex point, or apply any oils or creams to the feet prior to a reflexology treatment session. An oily foot makes direct contact with these tiny reflex points in the feet impossible.
- We *never* use any wooden probes, electrical stimulating devices, or anything of a mechanical or similar nature.

Reflexology is a simple science and is popular because of its simplicity. Nothing ever replaces the touch of the human hand.

The movement takes time to acquire because it is unusual for the thumb to work in this way. If you can visualise an old-fashioned pin cushion with the pins distributed throughout at intervals of about a quarter of an inch (0.6cm), you are going to bend your thumb and press the pin down into the pin cushion, go to the next pin and do likewise – tiny, tiny movements make the whole treatment far more successful, combined with a slow, deliberate movement, travelling over the whole surface of the foot.

We do not at any time work backwards, always an ongoing, forward creeping movement. Acquiring sufficient pressure takes time – time to build up sufficient muscle power in your thumb and index finger; after all, your thumbs have never been called on to work in this way before.

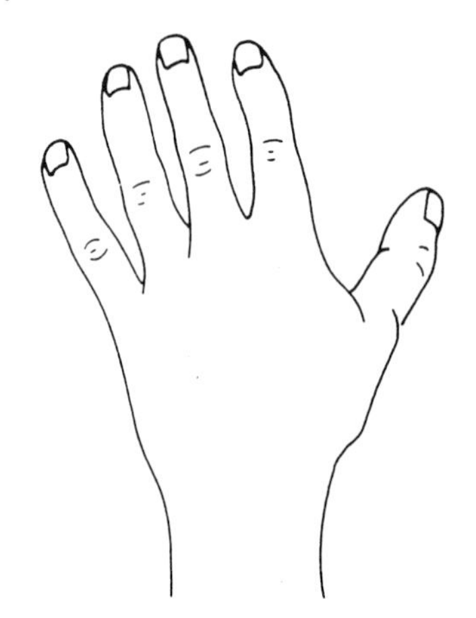

Figure 3.9 The thumb technique

CHAPTER 4 The digestive system

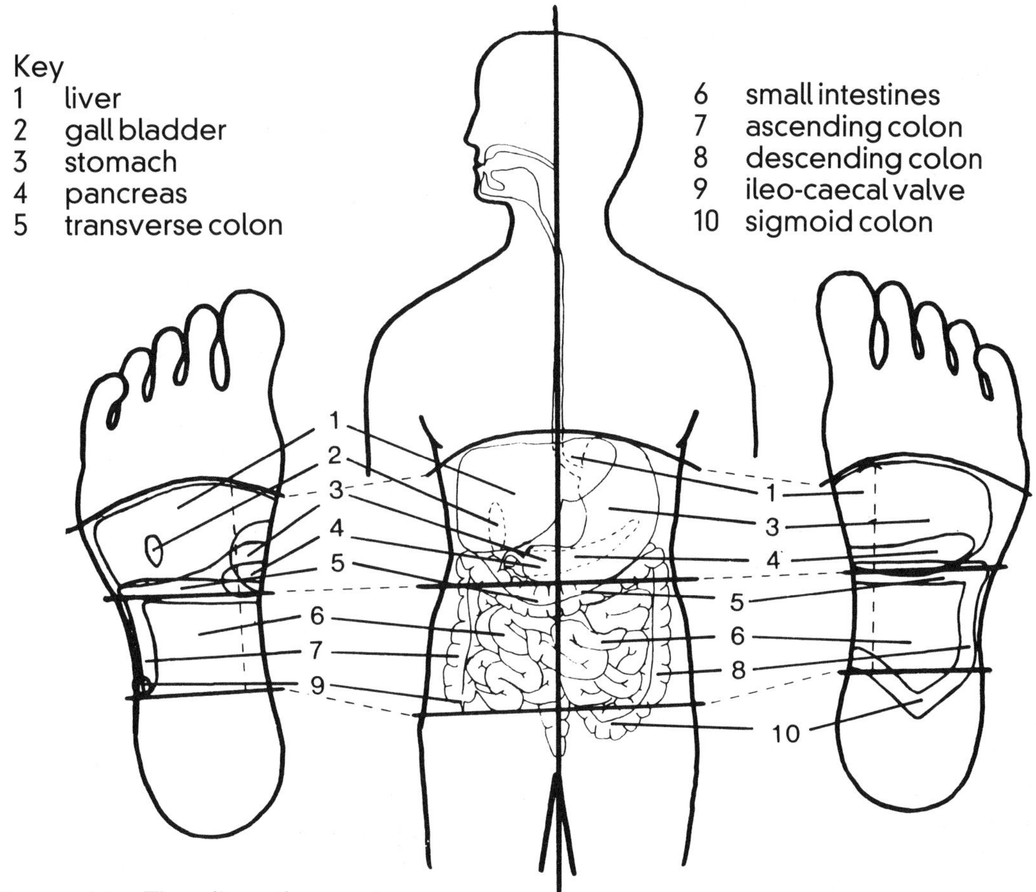

Figure 4.1 The digestive system

The digestive system is the term used to describe the digestive processes which take place at different levels in the alimentary canal to prepare food for absorption in the body. The alimentary tract is a long tube through which food is digested and absorbed. The process begins at the mouth and terminates at the anus. The various organs have distinctive names although structurally they are remarkably similar. The main ones are the mouth, pharynx, oesophagus, stomach, liver, small intestine, large intestine, rectum and the anal canal. The complex digestive processes gradually simplify the food we eat until it is in a form suitable for absorption. The activities in the digestive system can be placed under four main headings:

1 ingestion (taking food into the mouth);

2 chewing and swallowing (the mechanical breakdown of food in the mouth);

3 mixing and churning of the food by the stomach (breaking down the food into soluble compounds);

4 absorption and elimination by the intestines.

Food substances which have been eaten but cannot be digested and absorbed are excreted by the bowel as faeces.

The liver

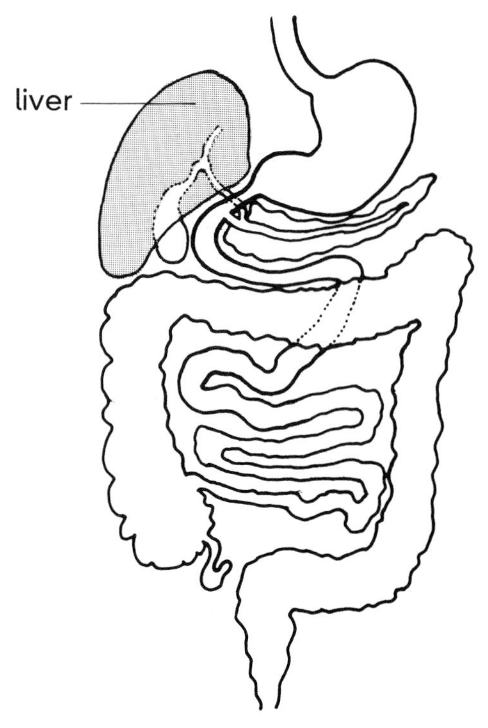

Figure 4.2

The liver is the largest gland in the body and weighs between 1 and 2.3kg. It is situated in the upper part of the abdominal cavity. The liver has four lobes, the two most obvious being the large right lobe and the smaller, wedge-shape left lobe. The other two, the caudate and quadrate lobes, are areas on the posterior surface. The lobes of the liver are made up of tiny lobules just visible to the naked eye.

Functions

1. It produces bile.
2. It deaminates amino acids.
3. It breaks down proteins to form uric acid which is excreted in the urine.
4. It is a regulator of the blood-glucose level. When the level of glucose becomes too high, the liver converts the excess into glycogen; and when the level becomes too low, the liver converts the appropriate amount of glycogen to glucose.
5. It desaturates fats – that is, it converts stored fats into a form which can be used by the tissues to provide energy.
6. It provides heat – the liver uses a considerable amount of energy, and has a high metabolic rate and produces a great deal of heat. It is the main heat-producing organ of the body.
7. It secretes bile. The liver cells synthesise constituents of bile from the mixed arterial and venous blood. These include bile salts, bile pigments and cholesterol. The bile consists in part of waste products from the breakdown of the red blood cells.
8. It stores vitamin B12, fat-soluble vitamins A, D, E and K, water-soluble vitamins riboflavin, niacin, pyridoxine, folic acid, iron and copper.
9. It synthesises vitamin A from carotene, the pro-vitamin found in some plants, such as carrots and the green leaves of vegetables.
10. It synthesises non-essential amino acids, plasma proteins and most of the blood-clotting factors from the available amino acids.
11. It detoxifies drugs and noxious substances such as toxins produced by microbes.
12. It metabolises poisons in alcoholic drinks.
13. It deactivates hormones, including insulin, cortisol, aldosterone, thyroid and sex hormones.

The gall bladder

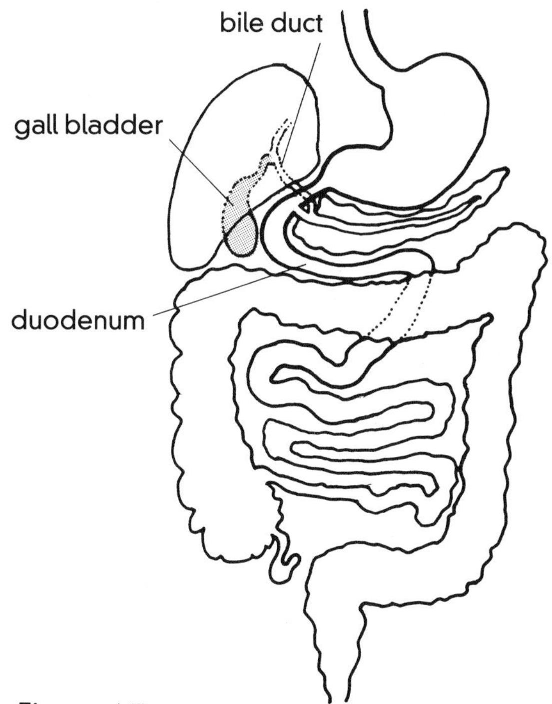

Figure 4.3

The gall bladder is a pear-shaped sac attached to the posterior surface of the liver by connective tissue. It has a fundus or expanded end, a body or main part, and a neck, which is continuous with the cystic duct.

Functions

1. It acts as a reservoir for bile.
2. The lining membrane adds mucus to the bile.
3. It absorbs water and is 10 to 15 times more concentrated than liver bile.
4. By the contraction of the muscular walls, bile is expelled from the gall bladder and passes via the bile ducts into the duodenum, to be used in the digestive process of fats. It also neutralises the acidity of chyme from the stomach.

The stomach

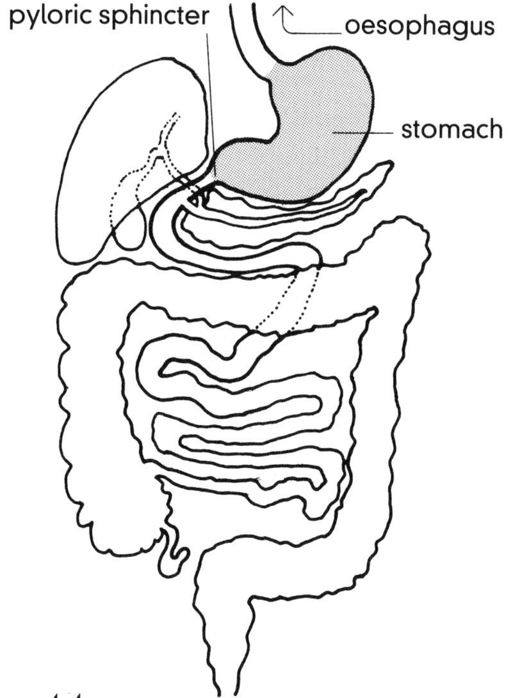

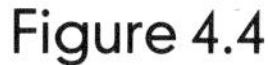

Figure 4.4

The stomach is a C-shaped dilated organ situated on the left side of the upper abdominal cavity. It has two curvatures: the lesser curvature is short, and lies on the posterior surface of the stomach and is the downward continuation of the posterior wall of the oesophagus. Just before the pyloric sphincter it bends upwards to complete the C-shape. The top of the stomach is referred to as the fundus. The main part is the body and the lower part, the pyloric antrum. When the stomach is inactive, the pyloric sphincter is relaxed and open, and when it contains food the sphincter is closed.

The stomach has three layers of smooth muscle fibres: the outer layer has longitudinal fibres; the middle layer has circular fibres; and the inner layer, oblique fibres. This arrangement allows for the churning and activation of the gastric activity as well as the peristaltic (clasping and compressing) movement. The fibres of the stomach vary with the amount of food it contains. When a meal has been eaten the food accumulates in the stomach in layers, the last part of the meal remaining in the fundus for some time.

Gastric juice

The mixing of a meal with gastric juices takes place very gradually. Gastric muscle contraction consists of churning movements that break down the bolus, mixing it with gastric juice, and peristaltic waves that propel the stomach contents towards the pylorus.

Gastric juice is secreted by special secretory glands and consists of water, mineral salts, mucus, hydrochloric acid, intrinsic factor, enzymes, and pepsinogen secreted by peptic cells in the glands.

Functions

1 Ptyalin starts the digestive process of carbohydrates in the mouth, being mixed with the saliva produced by the salivary glands. Water further liquidises the food swallowed.

2 Hydrochloric acid acidifies the food and stops the action of ptyalin.

3 The juices kill many microbes which may be harmful to the body.

4 They provide the acid environment needed for effective digestion by pepsin.

5 Pepsinogens are activated to pepsins by hydrochloric acid and by pepsins already present in the stomach.

6 Intrinsic factor (a protein compound) is necessary for absorption of vitamin B12.

7 Mucus prevents mechanical injury to the stomach wall by lubricating the contents and by protecting the stomach lining from the acid contents.

The small intestine

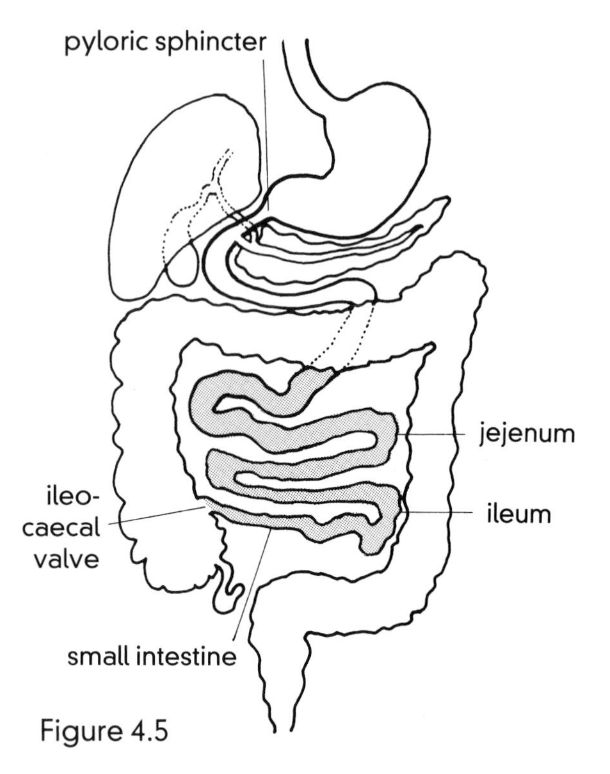

Figure 4.5

The small intestine continues from the stomach at the pyloric sphincter and leads into the large intestine at the ileo-caecal valve. It is a little over 5 metres long and lies in the abdominal cavity surrounded by the large intestine. In the small intestine, the digestion of food is completed and most of the absorption of nutrient materials take place. It consists of three parts:

- The **duodenum** which is about 25cm long curves around the head of the pancreas. At its mid-point there is an opening common to the pancreatic duct and the bile duct.
- The **jejunum** which is the middle part of the small intestine is about 2 metres long.
- The **ileum** or terminal part which is about 3 metres long ends at the ileo-caecal valve,

which controls the flow of material from the ileum to the large intestine and prevents regurgitation. About 3 litres of intestinal juice is secreted daily by the glands of the small intestine.

Functions

1 Onward movement of its contents, which is produced by peristaltic pendular movements.
2 Secretion of intestinal juice.
3 Completion of digestion of carbohydrates, protein and fats.
4 Protection against infection by microbes.
5 Secretion of hormones.
6 Absorption of nutrient material through the enormous surface area created by villi lining the intestine.

Digestion in the small intestine

When acid chyme passes into the small intestine it is mixed with pancreatic juice, bile and intestinal juice. In the small intestine the digestion of all the nutrients is completed.

Large intestine, rectum and anal canal

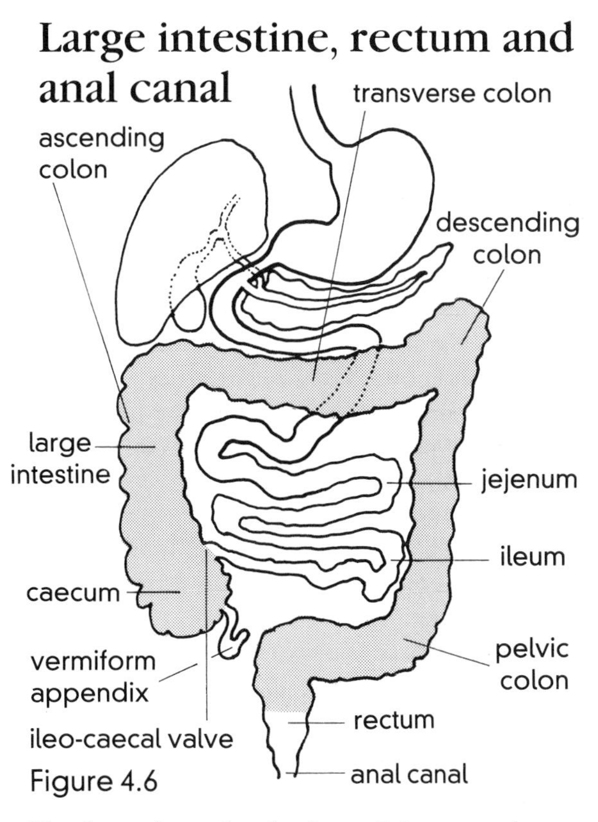

Figure 4.6

The large intestine is about 1.5 metres long, beginning at the caecum and terminating at the rectum and anal canal, deep in the pelvis. The space it encloses is larger than that of the small intestine. It forms an arch around the small intestine. The intestine is divided into the caecum, ascending colon, transverse colon, descending colon, sigmoid or pelvic colon, rectum and anal canal.

The caecum is the first part of the colon. It is a dilated portion which has a blind end inferiorly and is continuous with the ascending colon superiorly. Just below the junction of the two, the ileo-caecal valve opens from the ileum. The vermiform appendix is a fine tube closed at one end which leads from the caecum. It is usually about 13cm long and has the same structure as the walls of the colon but contains more lymphoid tissue.

The ascending colon passes up from the caecum to the level of the liver where it bends acutely to the left to become the transverse colon.

The transverse colon is a loop of colon which extends across the abdominal cavity in front of the jejunum and the stomach to the area of the spleen where it forms the left coeliac flexure (splenic flexure) by bending acutely downwards to become the descending colon.

The descending colon passes down the left side of the abdominal cavity, then curves towards the mid-line. After it enters the true pelvis, it is known as the pelvic colon. The pelvic colon, or sigmoid, is an S-shaped curve in the pelvis, which continues downwards to become the rectum.

The rectum is a slightly dilated part of the colon which is about 13cm long. It leads from the pelvic colon (sigmoid) and terminates in the anal canal.

The anal canal is a short canal about 3.8cm long in the adult, and leads from the rectum to the exterior. There are two sphincter muscles which control the anus. The internal sphincter, consisting of smooth muscle fibres, is under the control of the autonomic nervous system, and the external sphincter, formed by striated muscle, is under voluntary control.

Functions

The contents of the ileum, which pass through the ileo-caecal valve into the caecum, are fluid, even though some water has been absorbed in the small intestine. In the large intestine, absorption of water continues until the familiar semi-solid consistency of faeces is achieved.

Mineral salts, vitamins and some drugs are also absorbed into the blood capillaries from the large intestine. Gases in the bowel, which consist of some of the constituents of air, and many nitrogens swallowed with food and drink, are a feature of some anxiety states. Hydrogen, carbon dioxide and methane are produced by bacterial fermentation of an absorbed nutrient, especially carbohydrates. Gases pass out of the bowel as flatus. Large numbers of microbes are present in the faeces.

The pancreas

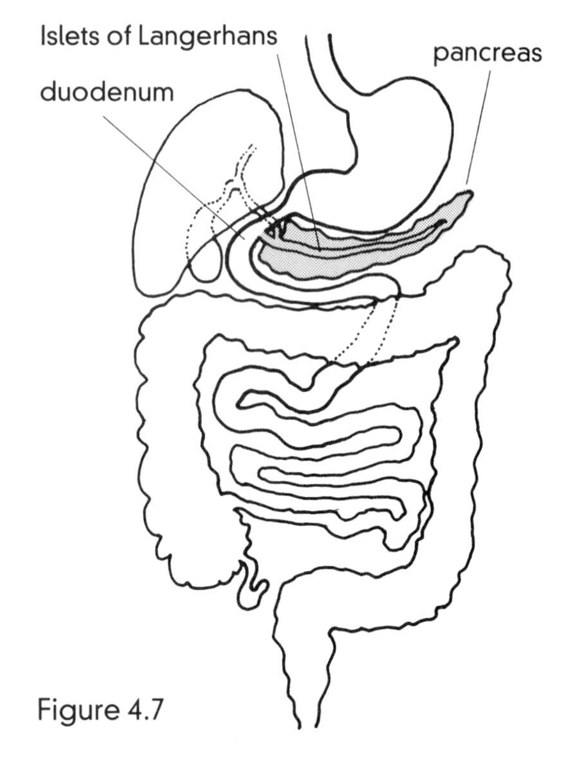

Figure 4.7

The pancreas is a pale grey gland, about 12 to 15cm long, which is situated near the epigastric region of the abdominal cavity. It consists of a broad head, a body and a narrow tail. The head lies in the curve of the duodenum, the body behind the stomach, and the tail lies in front of the left kidney and just reaches the spleen. The abdominal aorta and the inferior vena cava lie behind the gland.

The **Islets of Langerhans** are the endocrine areas of the pancreas. The alpha cells secrete glucagon and the beta cells produce insulin. These hormones work in opposition to control the glucose blood-sugar level. Inadequate production of insulin results in the disease diabetes mellitus.

The remainder of the pancreas produces pancreatic juice containing enzymes secreted in an alkaline juice which are released into the duodenum via the pancreatic duct to help in the digestive process of carbohydrates, proteins and fats.

Practical procedures for working the digestive system

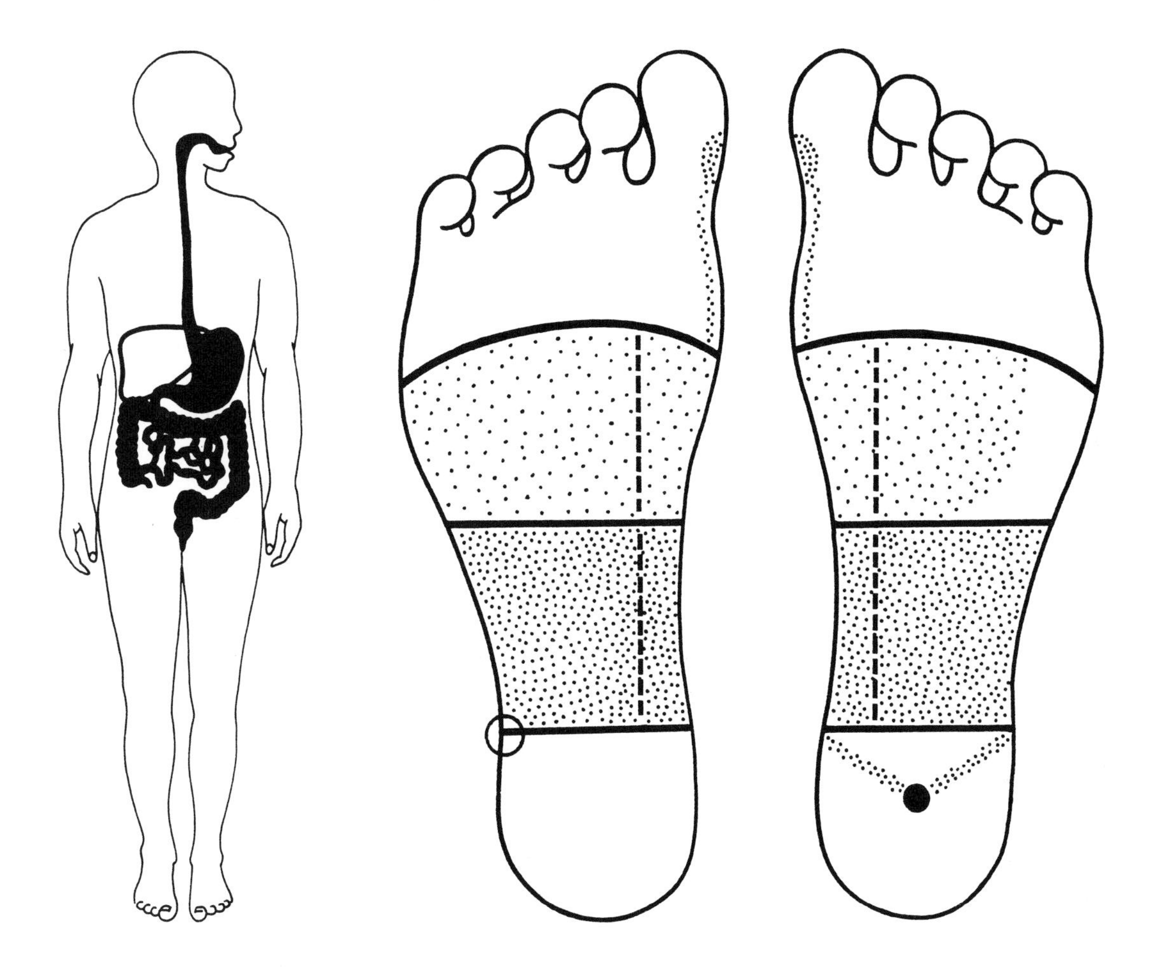

Figure 4.8 Areas relating to the digestive system

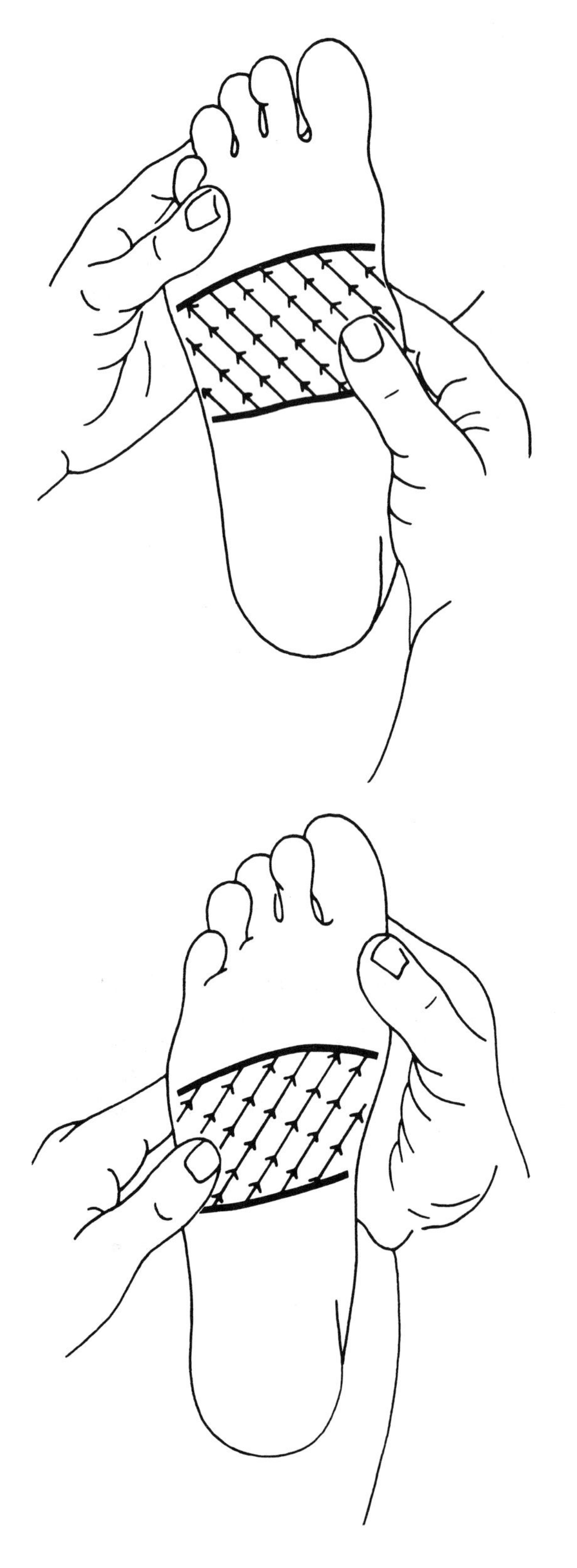

Figure 4.9 Working the liver area (right foot), zones 1 2 3 4 5, medial to lateral. Supporting the right foot with your left hand and using the right thumb, work out the entire area in a criss-cross direction from the medial to the lateral edge.

Figure 4.10 Working the liver area (right foot), lateral to medial.
Supporting the right foot with your right hand and using the left thumb, work out the entire area in a criss-cross direction from lateral to medial.

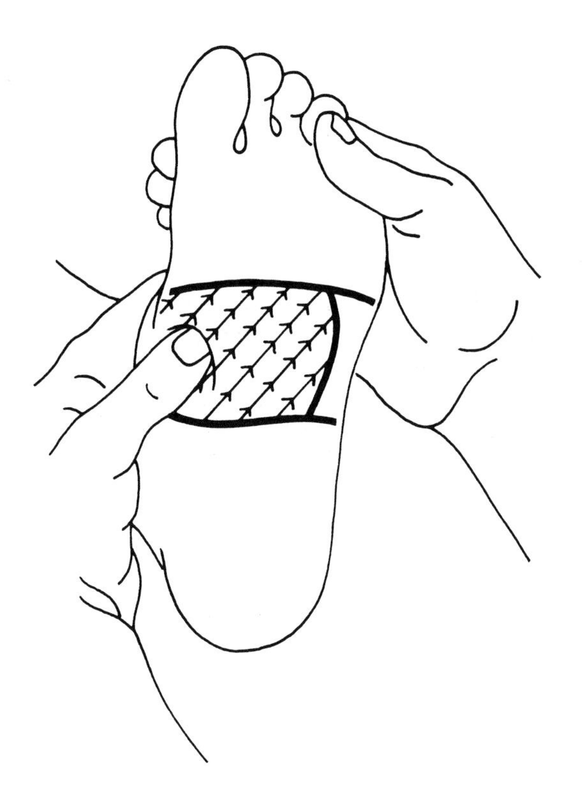

Figure 4.11 The stomach and pancreas (left foot), zones 1 2 3 4, medial to lateral. Supporting the left foot with your right hand and using the left thumb, work out the area in a criss-cross direction from medial to lateral.

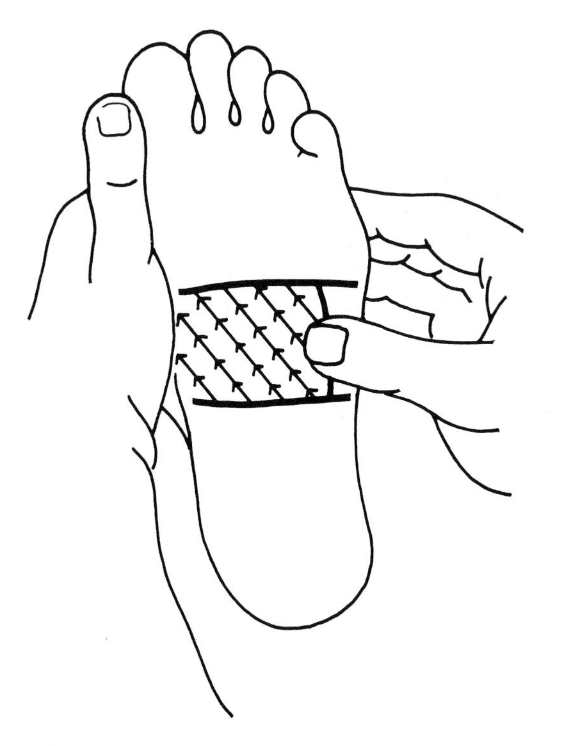

Figure 4.12 The stomach and pancreas (left foot), lateral to medial. Supporting the left foot with your left hand and using the right thumb, work out the area in a criss-cross direction from lateral to medial.

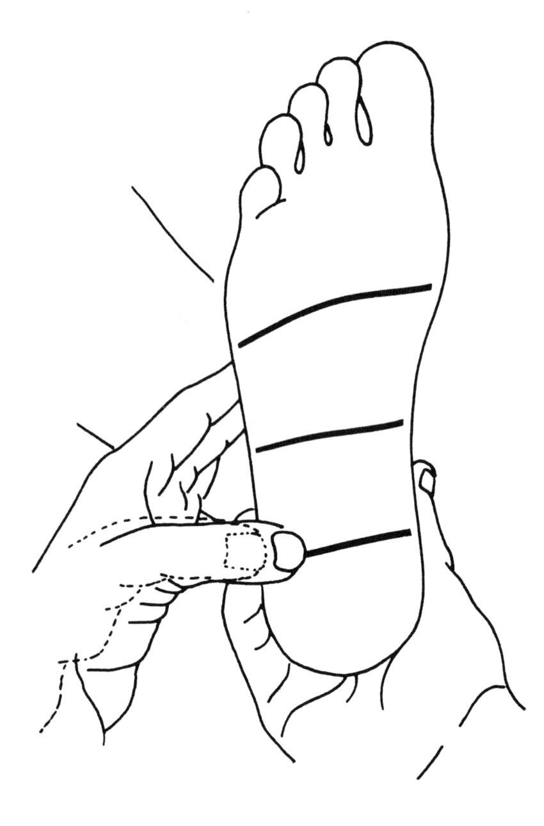

Figure 4.13 The ileo-caecal valve (right foot), zone 5, lateral – hooking out technique.
Supporting the right foot at the base of the heel with your right hand, place the left thumb on the heel line and use a 'hooking-out' procedure.

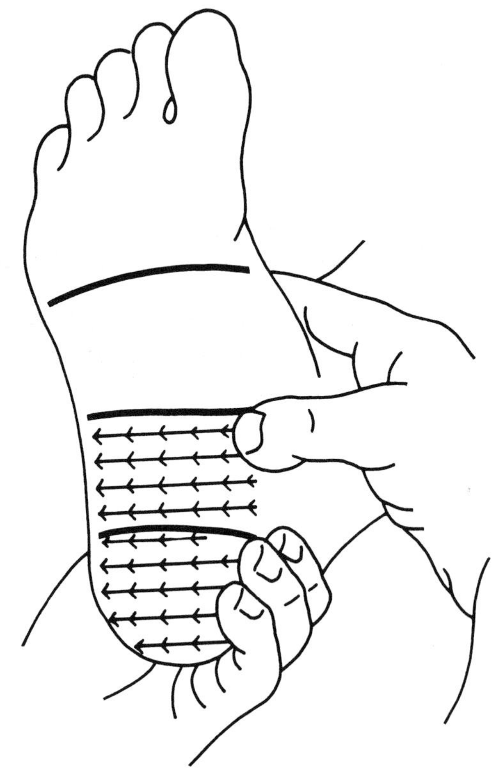

Figure 4.14 Intestinal area (right foot), zones 1 2 3 4 5, working out the whole of the intestinal area (ascending transverse and small intestines, buttock and back of pelvis).
Supporting the right foot at the base with your left hand, use the right thumb and work in straight lines across the foot from medial to lateral.

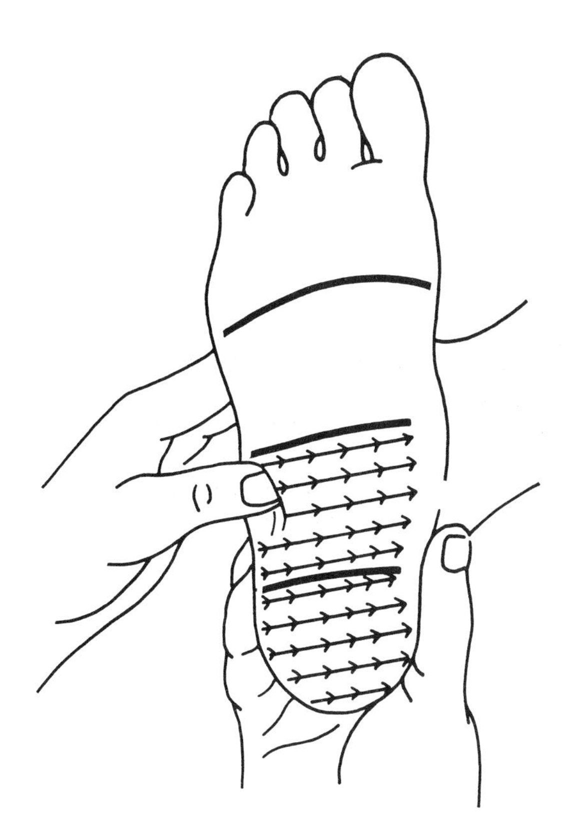

Figure 4.15 Intestinal area (right foot), zones 1 2 3 4 5, lateral to medial.
Supporting the right foot at the base with your right hand and using the left thumb, work out in straight lines from lateral to medial.

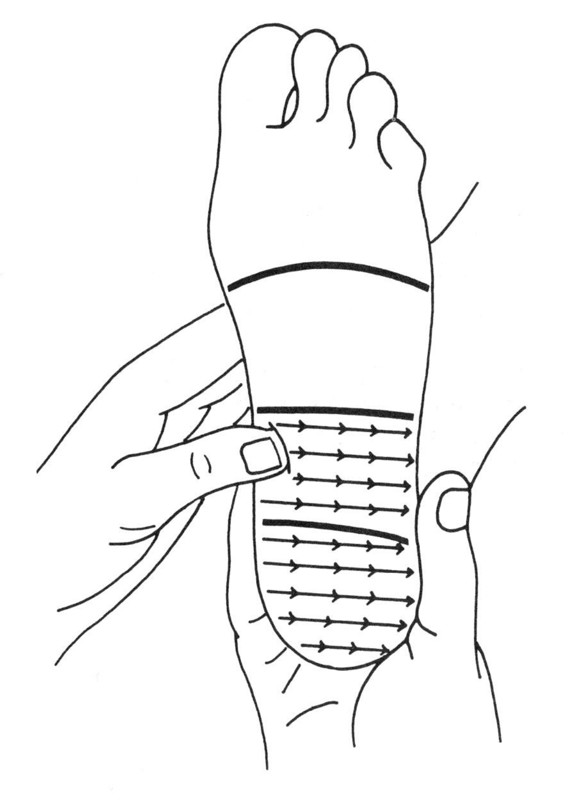

Figure 4.16 Intestinal area (left foot), zones 1 2 3 4 5, transverse descending and small intestines.
Supporting the left foot in your right hand at the base and using the left thumb, work out in straight lines from medial to lateral.

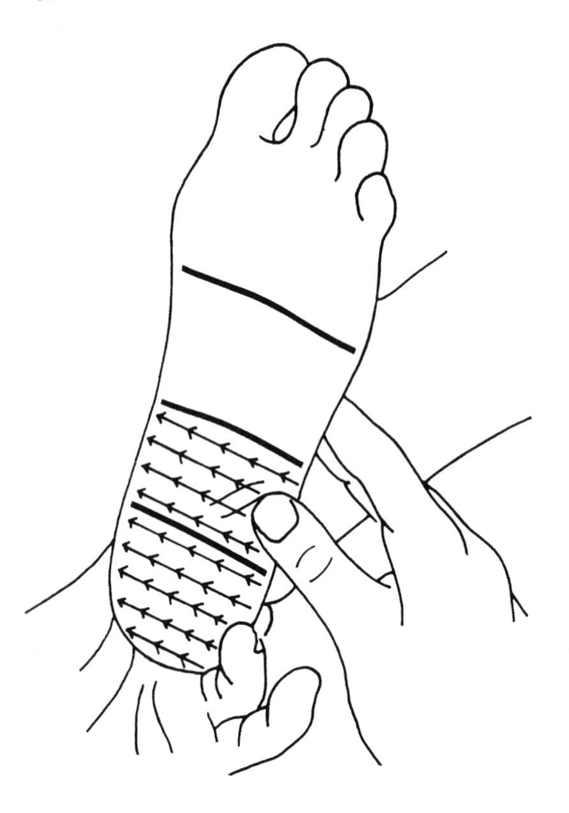

Figure 4.17 Intestinal area (left foot), zones 1 2 3 4 5, transverse descending and small intestines, including the buttock and back of the pelvis which are situated below the heel line.
Supporting the left foot at the base with your left hand and using the right thumb, work across in straight lines from lateral to medial.

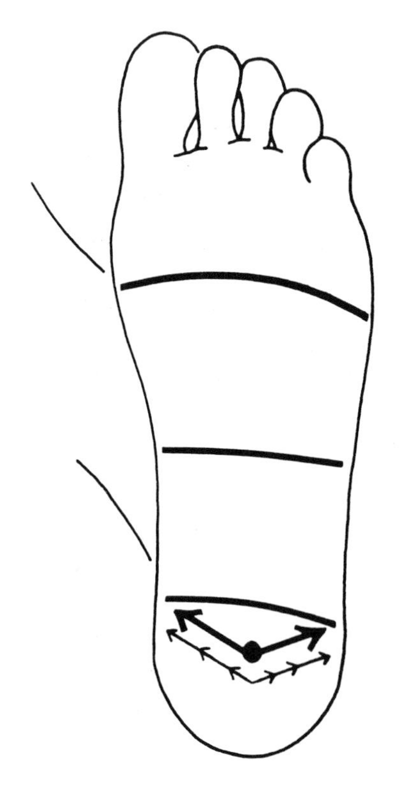

Figure 4.18 Area to sigmoid or pelvic colon, the bend (left foot), zone 3.
Supporting the left foot at the base with your left hand, place the right thumb on the mid point and work towards the medial edge.
Change direction and support the foot at the base with your right hand and work with the left thumb towards the lateral.

Case study: Irritable bowel syndrome

Malcolm came to me with a history of frequent diarrhoea and severe abdominal pain and total lethargy. He had been treated by the hospitals with the conventional progressive treatments starting with various antiacids and antibiotics in an attempt to control the excessive attacks of diarrhoea, but over the previous three years his condition had worsened so seriously that the only other treatment available was to resort to the use of steroids. Steroids are used to reduce the inflammation in the intestines but gave him little relief. Over a period of time he began to suffer severe effects from the high dosages of steroids.

In particular, he had noticed a very bloating effect of his face, occasional feelings of aggressiveness which were out of character, severe bruising if the slightest knock occurred, and an enhanced growth of hair on his body.

He was only 29 when he came to me and was rather despairing at the prospect of a lifetime with this routine of treatment to follow, which was obviously only controlling the disease and not curing it. I treated Malcolm over a period of three months and he attended for weekly treatments and was a very enthusiastic patient who took any advice that I was able to offer.

On commencing the treatment, I quite expected not to find any relative sensitivity in the feet due to the steroids. Normally, when a patient is undergoing treatment by steroids in some uncanny way it seems to depress the vitality of the body, resulting in an insensitivity in areas of the feet. However, knowing that whether Malcolm could feel the sensitivity or not the treatment would still work,

I proceeded to work on the areas of his feet which I knew should be super-sensitive, and these were of course the intestinal area and the entire digestive system. I gave him a complete treatment session, first, as is always the rule, concentrating on the sensitive areas that I knew would be damaged and weakened in his body.

He had consulted his own doctor and decided himself that he was going to try and reduce the amount of steroids he was taking and try another form of approach to improve his very poor health. The doctor was quite co-operative and suggested that only a very small reduction in the steroids should be made initially, and so we proceeded with the treatment sessions.

Malcolm's first indication of any improvement was when he was able to reduce his steroids to half and still not have any unpleasant symptoms. He felt a general lightness, a sense of well-being and relaxation which he had not experienced for many years and a hope that this treatment was going to lead him towards better health for the future.

Malcolm did so well with reflexology that within two months he had removed himself from the steroids completely and found that in fact his symptoms did not return. He regained one stone in weight within four months. He had only occasional bouts of diarrhoea which very quickly subsided and enjoyed a tremendous improvement in his general health. With this renewed vigour he was able to return to his full-time job, take up some passive forms of exercise and, most important of all, his wife was so impressed by the benefits of reflexology that she became a practitioner.

CHAPTER 5 The respiratory system

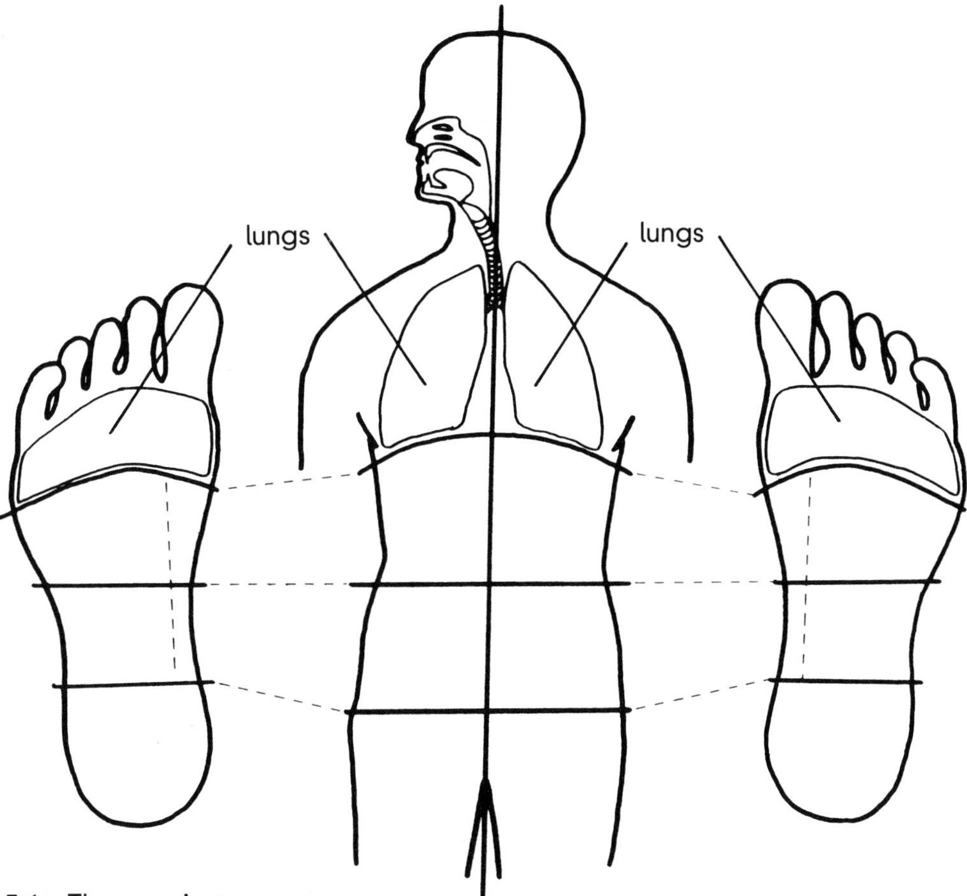

Figure 5.1 The respiratory system

The respiratory system involves two spongy bags, the lungs, occupying most of the chest cavity. Muscles work the lungs like bellows and an air tube links the lungs to the nose and mouth. Air breathed in through the nose or through the mouth grows warm and moist on passing through the nasal passages and pharynx. Air continues down the windpipe or trachea except when it is shut off by the epiglottis as you swallow. Air then passes through two bronchi to the lungs. Inside the lungs, bronchi branch out into small tubes called bronchioles. Bronchioles end in alveolar sacs, clusters of tiny chambers known as alveoli. Spread flat, the alveoli in a pair of lungs would cover half a tennis court. Their thin walls support a network of capillaries, the tiny tubes containing blood. Gaseous interchange takes place in the alveolar sacs of the lungs. Air is inhaled, and oxygen, carbon dioxide and waste products extracted, passing into the blood through a network of fine capillaries. The respiratory system involves air going into and coming out of the body. The system supplies body cells with oxygen for burning food to produce energy. The lungs are operated by the diaphragm muscle, which is a large sheet of muscle below the lungs, and by muscles that move the ribs up and down called intercostal muscles.

As you breathe in, the ribs move up and out and the diaphragm moves down to give an elongation to the chest cavity. This expands the chest cavity and draws air into the lungs. Breathing out, the ribs move down and in and the diaphragm moves up. This contracts the chest cavity and forces air out of the lungs. Sounds are created by special structures in the body's airway. Exhaled air flows through the larynx or the voice box, a broad part of the upper windpipe protected by tough cartilage that forms the Adam's apple. Two bands of tissue called 'vocal cords' form a V-shaped opening across the larynx. As we speak, these tighten, narrowing the opening. Exhaled air vibrates the cords and produce sounds; the longer the cords, the higher the pitch. Sounds vary with different positions of the tongue, lips and teeth. The nasal cavity gives resonance to the voice.

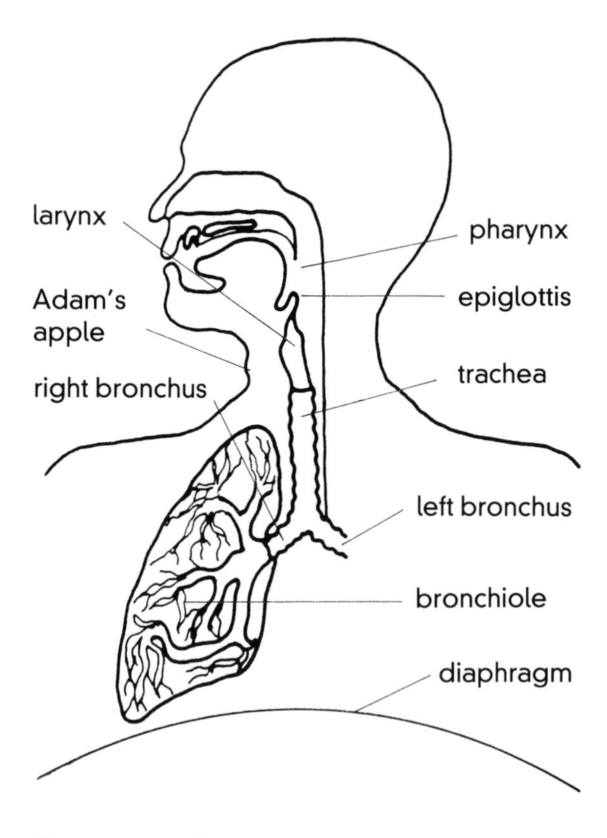

Figure 5.2 The respiratory organs

Conditions benefiting from reflexology

The types of conditions that the reflexologist will be able to relieve and assist are bronchitis, asthma, emphysema and all the upper respiratory tract infections, which will be covered in Chapter 10, on the sinus areas and the face. Problems in the respiratory system often have their root cause in digestion, and it may be difficult for you to accept that in order to get good relief from a respiratory condition the digestive system needs to be worked, but this is true. There is evidence that because infants with an immature digestive system, and who also have a family history of illness such as asthma, hay fever, bronchitis, and so on, are introduced too soon to a wide variety of foods, respiratory problems often start in their early years. Babies, who after all, are born without teeth, were really not meant to have any food other than breast milk until they had grinding teeth, but these do not appear until the second year. The fashion was to feed very small infants, about six weeks old, on high-protein cereals and dairy products. This can cause stress to the digestive system and an irritation in the stomach lining, and result in the child having episodes of infection in the upper and lower respiratory tracts. The most common route that such infections take is inner-ear conditions in the first four months of life, followed by constant catarrh, and if this routine continues then the child often exhibits symptoms which doctors refer to in the early stages as 'wheezy bronchitis'. It is then that the treatment of constant bottles of antibiotics is started to control infection. Antibiotics have quite a disastrous effect on the intestine. In fact, they destroy the flora, which are the friendly bacteria which keep the intestinal tract healthy, so again you are putting into an already immature digestive system drugs to control the repeated infections. It is essential to eliminate all dairy products and wheat-based cereal to give the digestive system a rest and allow it to mature during its normal course of time. If alteration to diet and frequent treatments of reflexology are undertaken, the overall results are normally exceptionally good.

Asthma

Asthma is increasing in today's society. There are various reasons for this. Among them dietary problems definitely form a large part, and so do all the colourings in drinks and food which cause irritation to the digestive system and to the delicate mucous membrane which lines the entire respiratory tract. These additives should be avoided. We also have problems due to double-glazing, central heating and fitted carpets, which all encourage dust mites to remain in the home and exacerbate the asthma. The draughty homes of the past allowed movement of air, and these mites were therefore controlled. We also have external environmental pollutions that irritate the nasal and lung passages. There are also crop sprays and the domestic sprays we use in our homes, as well as fumes from traffic both in the air and on the ground, which, among other things, add to air pollution.

Practical procedures for working the respiratory system

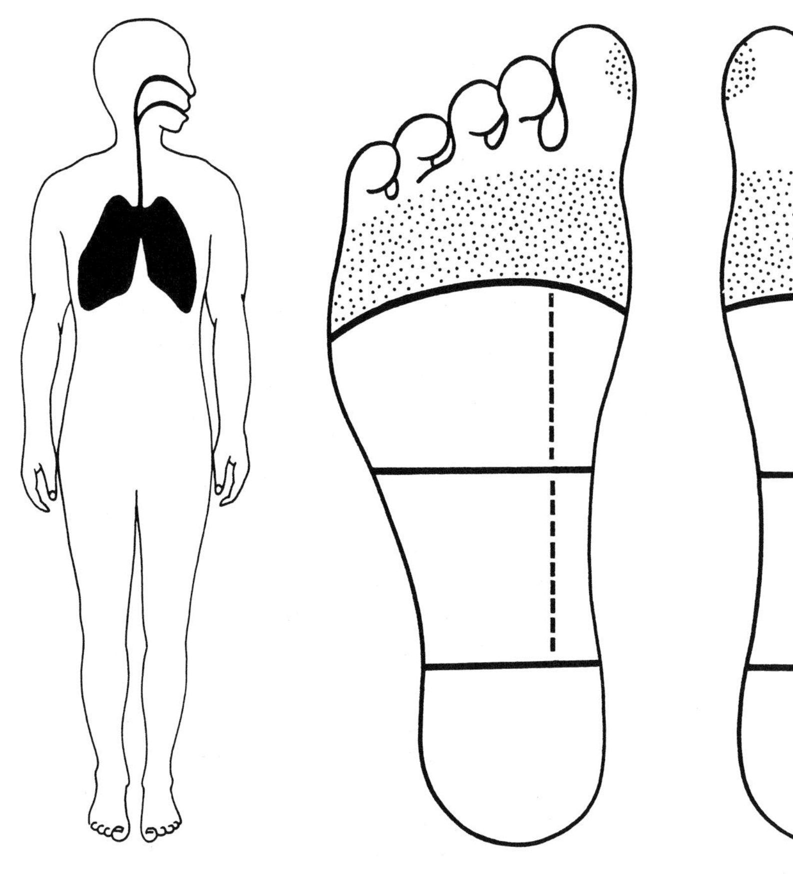

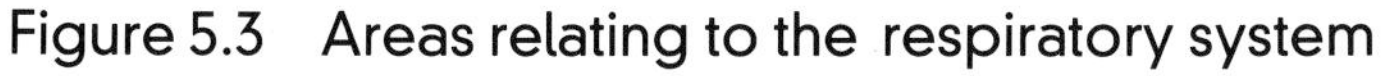

Figure 5.3 Areas relating to the respiratory system

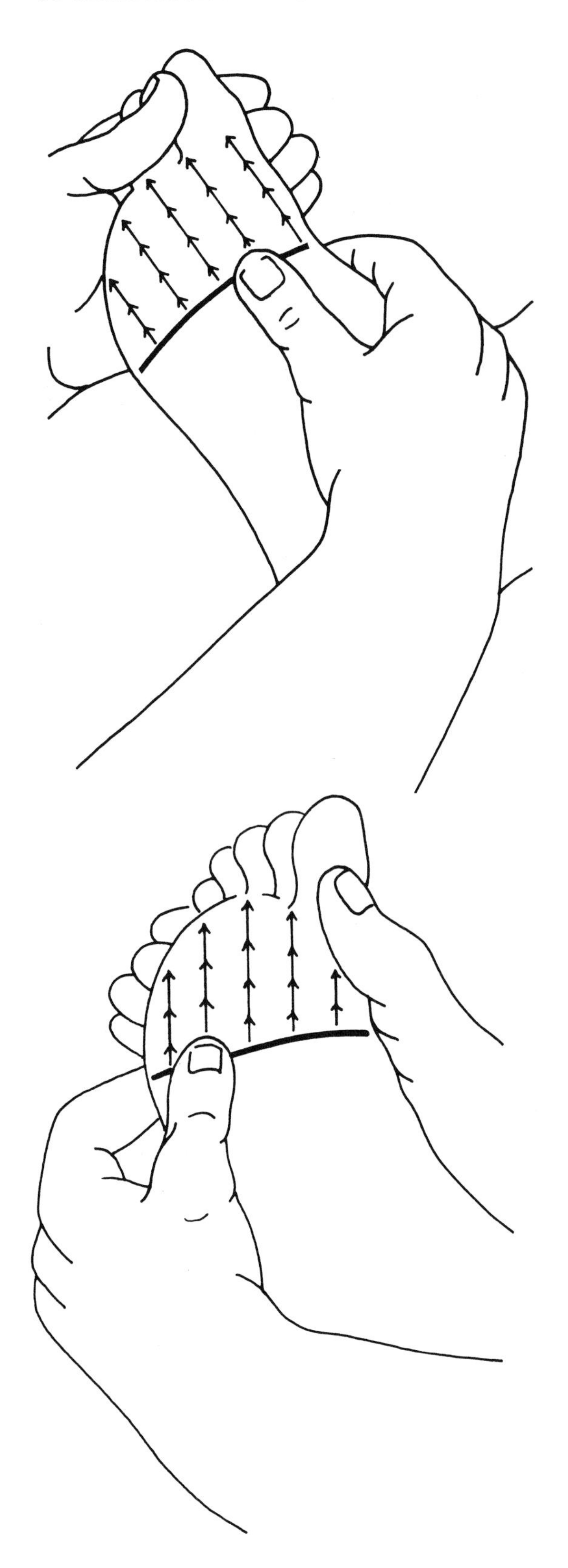

Figure 5.4 Working the lung area (right foot, plantar view), zones 1 2 3 4 5, medial to lateral.
Supporting the right foot with your left hand at the top and using the right thumb, work up the foot in straight lines from medial to lateral.

Figure 5.5 Working the lung area (right foot, plantar view), zones 1 2 3 4 5, lateral to medial.
Supporting the right foot with your right hand at the top and using the left thumb, work up the foot in straight lines from lateral to medial.

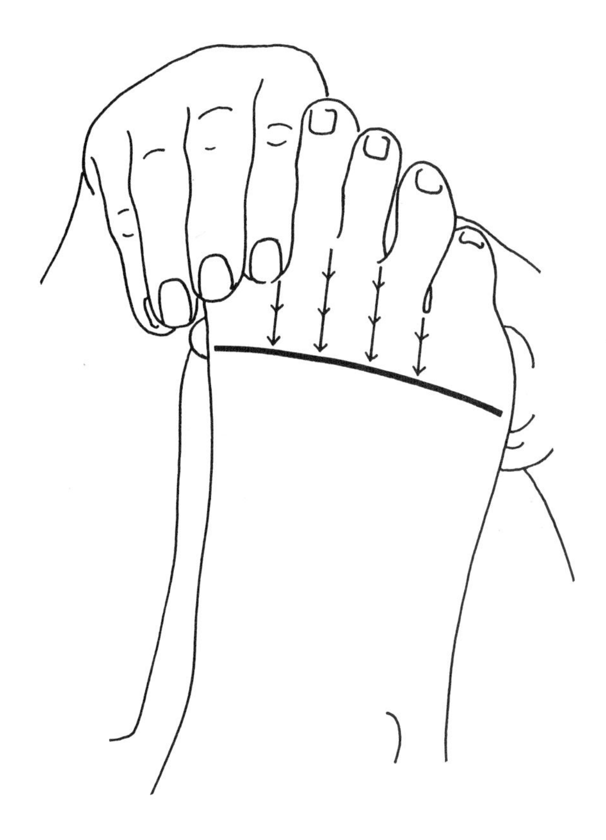

Figure 5.6 Working the lung/breast area (dorsal view), zones 1 2 3 4 5, medial to lateral.
Supporting the right foot with your left fist and using the right index finger, proceed downwards from medial to lateral.

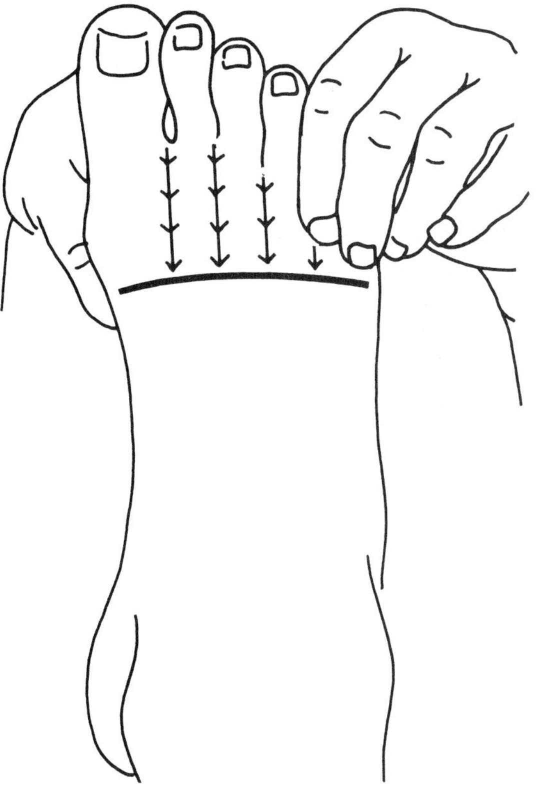

Figure 5.7 Working the lung/breast area (dorsal view), zones 1 2 3 4 5, lateral to medial.
Supporting the right foot with your right fist and using the left index finger, proceed downwards from lateral to medial.

Case study: Asthma

A case that I remember being extremely rewarding was a man of 50 who had been a sufferer with severe asthma since the age of 5. He rang to see whether I considered that any relief could be obtained for him after all these years. His asthma had been controlled by various inhalers, and in his acute stages he had had to resort to episodes of steroid treatment. He said that without his inhalers he was unable to follow his occupation and the quality of his life was extremely impaired.

I did treat him on a regular basis for about three months, and after the initial bad reaction to the first treatment when he did actually have an asthma attack which was quite severe, he then made a gradual improvement. At the end of the three-month period he was only using his inhaler on very rare occasions, which was amazing as it is so difficult to come off medication when you have been relying upon it for so many years. After the frequent treatments over the three-month period he attended on a monthly basis for another year, and at the end of that time said he had not felt so well in his life and only wished that he had sought out the support of a reflexologist in his earlier years.

Case study: Emphysema

I was called to treat a very sick man. He was the father of a patient of mine who had been attending my surgery for several months for treatment for her migraine. Her father was extremely ill with emphysema. In emphysema the lungs lose their elasticity because of the collapse of the alveolar walls, which greatly reduces their surface area for gaseous interchange to take place. The patient has difficulty in breathing out and becomes distressed, which causes air to be trapped in the diseased airways. The chest is elevated by the accessory muscles of respiration, and the diaphragm becomes flattened.

Medically, there is not a lot that can be done, apart from controlling the symptoms, which are serious, and this poor gentleman was almost disabled. Most of his life was spent sitting in a chair, as any exertion, just a walk across the room, caused such extreme breathlessness and exhaustion that he was unable to manage. He was on steroidal treatment to try and break down the excessive inflammation in his lungs and anti-diuretic tablets to try and control the water in his lung area. His heart was extremely large due to the excess work it had been involved in for many years.

The doctor obviously felt that the improvement this poor man might make would at best be minimal, but as the daughter of the patient was so anxious to try and do something for her father I agreed to see him. With his breathlessness, it was distressing to watch him struggle from the car into my surgery, which took a long time. The next hurdle was to get the patient on the couch, another physical effort which ended in extreme breathlessness and exhaustion.

The patient enjoyed the treatment session immensely, and said he felt very relaxed and had a feeling of ease around his diaphragm area.

The following day I telephoned him to see if he had had any adverse reactions. He said that in fact he was feeling well but noticed that there had been a very large increase in the amount of urine output. I felt that this was a beneficial sign and surely would give a lot of relief to the fluid levels in his lungs.

It was obviously not going to be a case where this man would receive a great benefit, but in fact the following two years before he died were much easier ones. He had far fewer episodes of admission to hospital, was able to do a few, very simple, household chores which gave him a feeling of self-worth, and all in all he and his family were very satisfied that reflexology had improved the quality of his life.

CHAPTER 6 The circulatory system

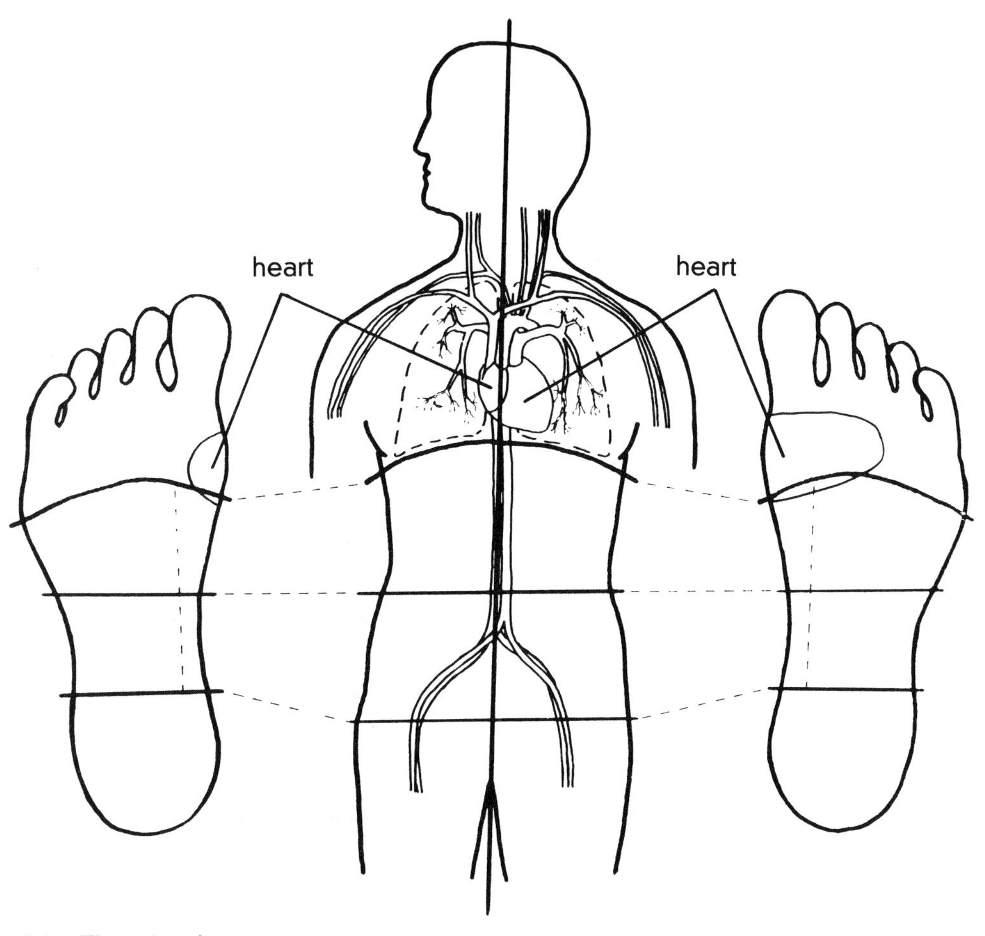

Figure 6.1 The circulatory system

The heart is a muscular pumping organ, which beats continuously in order to circulate blood around the body. The heart functions as two halves, each consisting of an atrium and a pumping centre, the ventricle. Each chamber is separated by a valve controlling the blood flow between chambers.

Deoxygenated blood enters the heart through the right atrium via the superior and inferior vena cava. Then the blood is forced through the tricuspid valve into the right ventricle. The blood is then pumped to the lungs via the pulmonary valve to the pulmonary artery.

Oxygenated blood from the lungs travels through the pulmonary veins to the left atrium, through the mitral valve to the left ventricle, and then leaves the heart through the aorta to be circulated around the body.

Nerve signals to the heart regulate its beat. Heart beats speed up during exercise as the heart pumps faster and harder to satisfy the body's extra needs for blood and oxygen.

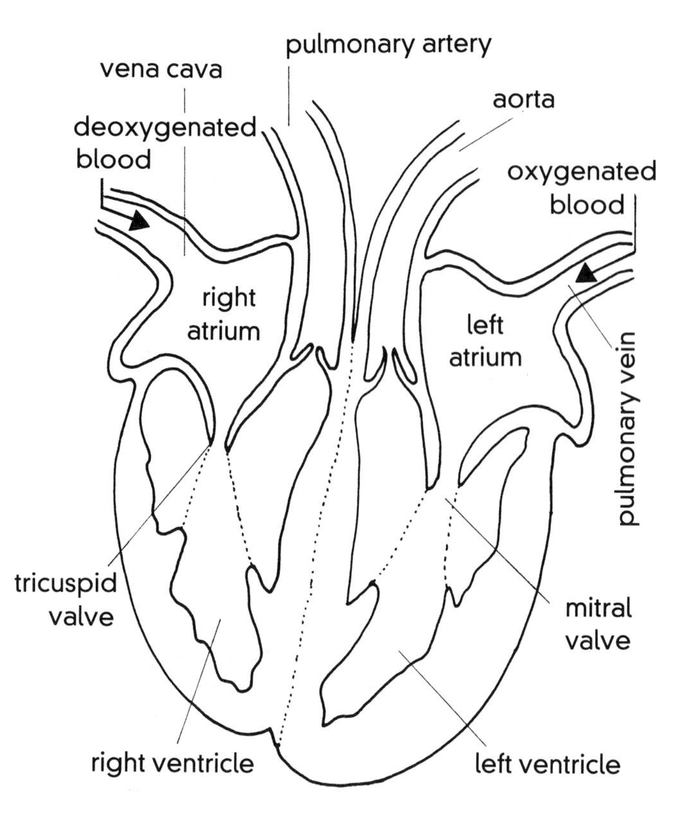

Figure 6.2 The heart

Arteries, veins and capillaries

Arteries are the largest blood vessels, carrying high-pressure, oxygenated blood away from the heart. They have thick, muscular walls, which branch into countless tiny tubes called arterioles.

Veins are large tubes that return low-pressure, deoxygenated blood to the heart. Veins have thinner walls than arteries. They are supplied with blood by tiny blood vessels called venules. The smallest of these are capillaries, which link arterioles and venules.

The heart's pumping action forces blood out through the arteries, arterioles and capillaries. Food and nutrients in the blood pass out through the capillary wall to nourish surrounding tissue.

From the capillaries, blood flows back to the heart, through the venules and veins. Muscles near veins keep the blood on the move, and the valves in the big veins stop blood flowing the wrong way.

Each heart beat sends a wave through your arteries. You can feel this if you place your finger on the underside of your forearm behind the base of your thumb. For most adults the pulse rate is about 70 per minute, but it is more rapid in children and slower in elderly people. Your pulse rate increases with exercise and also with emotion.

Blood pressure is the pressure exerted by blood on the artery walls. It varies with how fast and hard the heart beats and with the condition of arteries. You will see on page 45 the correct working procedure for working on the circulatory system.

Increase in heart disease

There has been a very large increase in coronary arterial disease; in fact, more and more younger males, in particular, are having heart and arterial surgery than ever before. This is due in the main to affluent living, the fast food routine which we have adopted in the western world and the lack of exercise over the years since the war due to the constant use of cars, escalators and lifts, and also the increase of a different sort of stress which is created by living in a rather complicated volume-packed society. The heart is a muscle, and needs to exercise regularly in order to act efficiently.

Females have a lower incident rate of heart disease due to the fact that during their menstrual years the output by the ovary of oestrogen and progesterone has great benefits in keeping the artery walls healthy. After the menopause the statistics of heart and arterial disease in females rises to join the same statistics as those of males.

Hormone replacement therapy is a very popular form of treating menopausal disorders and has been proven to decrease the likelihood of women getting circulatory diseases. This is simply because the oestrogen and progesterone levels are being maintained by taking hormones by mouth.

Conditions benefiting from reflexology

The types of conditions benefiting from reflexology are angina, irregular heart beat, known as tachycardia in its over-productive form and bradycardia in its latent form. Reflexology is also very beneficial for those who have suffered a heart attack. It can be of great support in the post-operative care of these patients.

Any form of circulatory malfunction can be improved with reflexology. Many patients report an improvement in circulation generally and cold feet often become a thing of the past. There are absolutely no dangers associated in treating any heart condition. If you accept that the heart is a muscle that is similar to other organs and muscles in the body, this then becomes a very safe and effective area to work on.

Reflexology is of tremendous benefit to diabetic sufferers who have increasing problems with circulatory disease during their later years. It is quite normal for a diabetic eventually to suffer coronary conditions. They are far more likely to have a stroke, renal failure, loss of sight, and unfortunately the blood supply to their legs is often severely diminished, and many suffer the disasters of gangrene. Reflexology has proved to be of great value to these sufferers and is highly recommended for diabetics of all age groups.

Areas to work for heart conditions

In heart conditions, the main areas to work in order to assist the patient are obviously the heart and the lung area. Diaphragm relaxation is of the utmost importance. It is also of great benefit to work the whole of the thoracic spine many times in order to stimulate the nerve supply to the whole thoracic cavity area. Working on the liver is very beneficial also.

I always find it strange that the heart is identified as an organ of romance. Hearts are portrayed on cards expressing feeling for our loved ones; we suffer a broken heart; we have heart-felt warm feelings towards our friends and relatives; we meet many cold-hearted people; and we are all aware of the stimulation of heart beat when we experience an emotional response to another person. If we look at the physical heart it shows nothing of any sentimental or attractive value. It is in fact just a large pump with lots of tubes arising out of it. Feelings we experience that we associate with our heart in times of happiness or grief are actually vibrations and stimulations from our solar plexus, which is a large nerve complexity behind the stomach. These stimulations and vibrations are felt in our heart area, and also the increased output of adrenaline stimulates heart beat.

Practical procedures for working the circulatory system

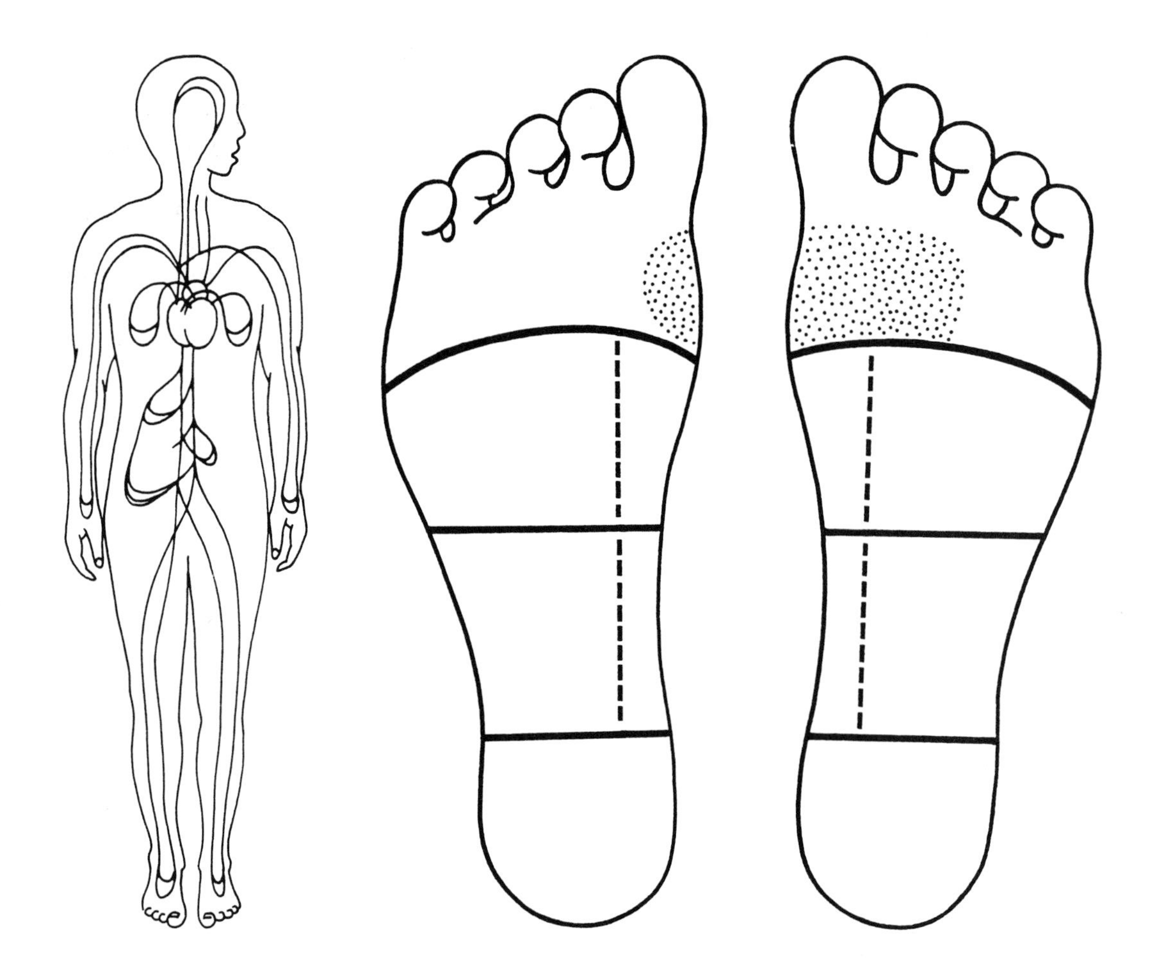

Figure 6.3 Areas relating to the circulatory system

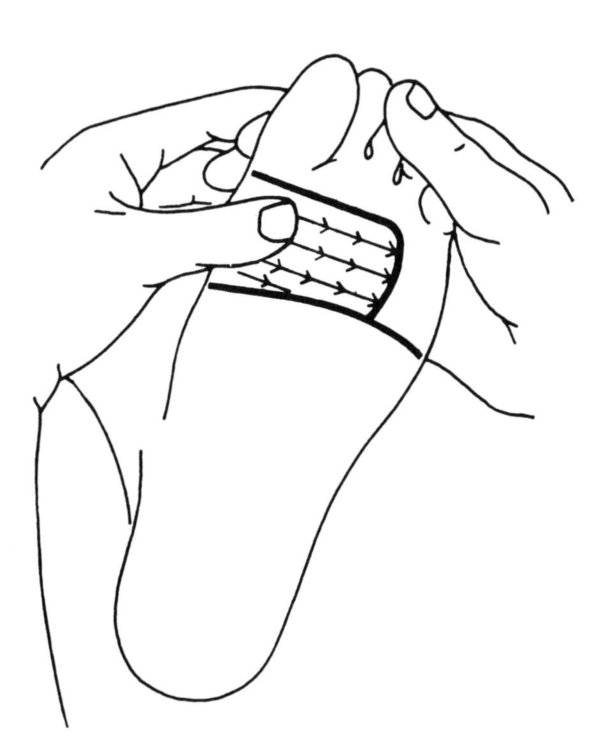

Figure 6.4 The heart (left foot), plantar view, zones 1 2 3, medial to lateral. Supporting the left foot with your right hand at the top and using the left thumb, work in horizontal lines.
As the heart area will already have been worked out thoroughly within the respiratory area we do not overwork this area and therefore need only to proceed in one direction.

Case study: Heart attack

I remember treating a patient who was only 38 when he suffered a massive heart attack. It had come completely out of the blue, as he had had no signs or symptoms of any heart condition before. Obviously, this episode came as a shock to him.

Norman was a very high-powered business executive; his job took him to all parts of the country and also to many others, so he spent a lot of his time travelling both by air and road. He admitted that his lifestyle was not particularly healthy – exercise had become a thing of the past – and he was inactive and spent too much time sitting down. He was frequently present at business meetings which took place at lunch time. These meals were always laced with an abundance of alcohol, and his drinking had definitely increased over the years.

His lifestyle had offered him many material gains, which he thought were most important. He had an enormous house, two or three large expensive cars, all his children were at private schools and he had quite a heavy entertaining commitment with his so-called friends.

He admitted that he was hardly aware of his children's existence; as his stays away from home were so frequent, in fact he hardly ever saw them, so communication levels were very limited.

His wife and he had grown apart over the years but he still felt that what he offered his family was of maximum importance and their lifestyle was able to put him at the top of the ladder as regard being a good husband and father.

Lying in bed in the intensive care unit with his life-threatening condition made him evaluate the life which he had mapped out for himself and he realised that maybe this heart attack was a sign that he must either change the direction of the road on which he was travelling or face very early demise. That he confided in me his fears and realisation that the life he had thought was so good was in fact of very little value was a positive way forward and he began having regular reflexology treatments.

In the early weeks after his discharge from hospital the exertion he had to make to just come in his car to my surgery and get onto the treatment couch was distressing. He was extremely breathless and weak, and said that he felt that all the life and energy had been drained from his body. He did in fact have to have three months' leave from his managerial position, and as he began to feel an improvement in his strength he started regular walking – a quarter of a mile the first week, then half a mile, increasing over the month to a mile on most days. He joined a relaxation class and was a very receptive patient who felt that reflexology had offered him a turning point to a new direction in his life.

He did in fact make an excellent recovery and had treatments, often twice weekly, with me. The three months' rest from his job gave him the opportunity to re-evaluate his needs, and he decided that the big country house and the three fast cars weren't really essential elements to happiness. His relationship with his children was second rate and his marriage certainly had lots of weak spots in it mainly due to his inability to 'give anything of any spiritual or emotional nature'.

Norman did actually leave his demanding job and took a far less stressful position. He accepted a large drop in his salary and it therefore became essential to move to a smaller house.

Because he heeded the warning signs that came into his life and changed the direction of things he is still alive today – ten years on. He has not had another heart attack and has no need to be on any form of medication.

He has a much richer life with his family, and says that his whole lifestyle is of greater benefit and enjoyment than ever it was before.

Norman was obviously one of the sensible ones; many people continue on the same unhealthy path and end up by having yet another and eventually a fatal heart attack.

CHAPTER 7 The lymphatic system

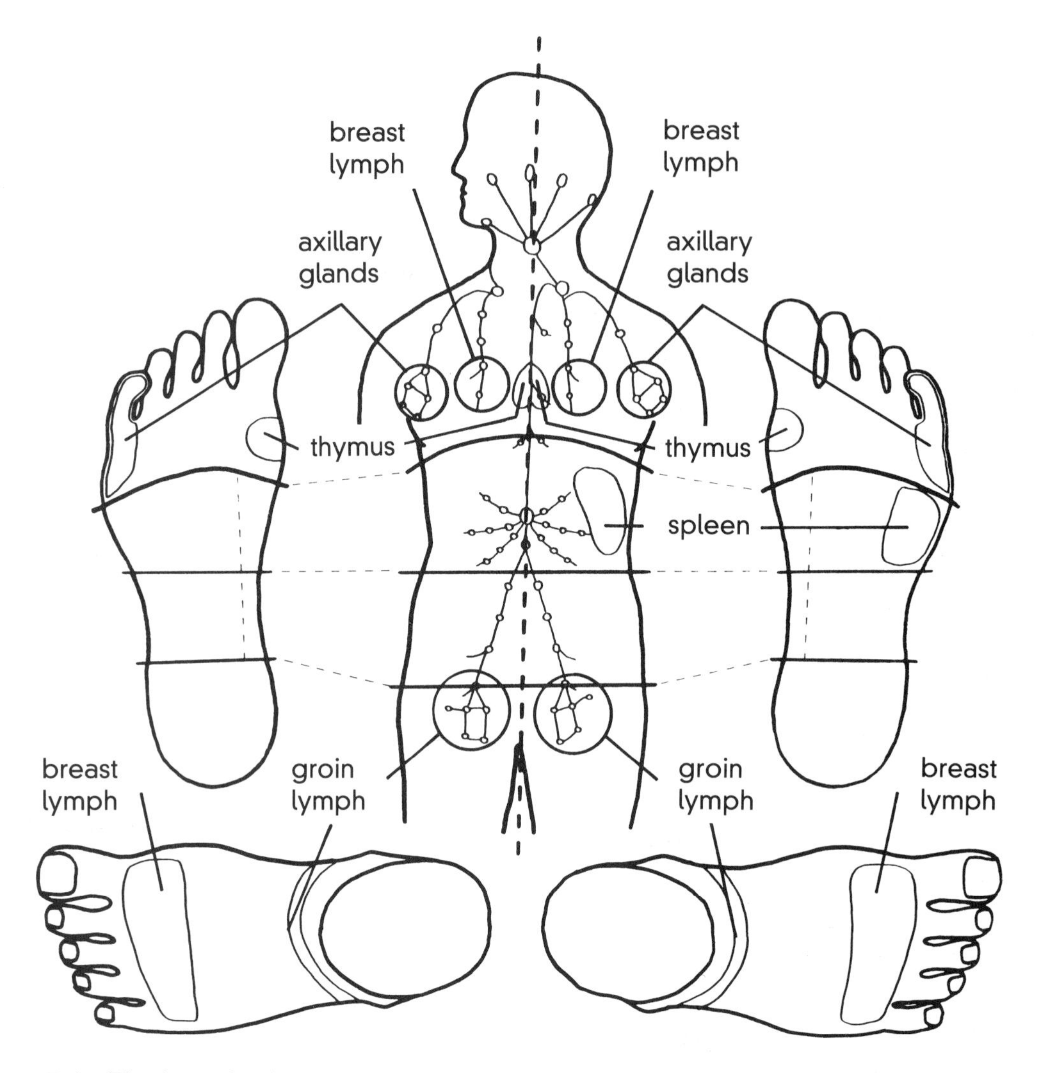

Figure 7.1 The lymphatic system

This is a network of vessels throughout the body that traps fluid escaped from blood vessels and returns it to the blood supply. The system also absorbs harmful bacteria and other dangerous substances.

It works by blood pressure forcing fluid from tiny blood vessels into surrounding tissues. Most fluid finds its way into these blood vessels, but some enters the lymph vessels. The fluid, now called lymph, flows towards the thoracic duct or to the right lymphatic duct. The forces that drive it are muscle activity and pulsating blood vessels. Valves in lymph vessels ensure that the lymph travels in only one direction. From the thoracic duct, lymph drains back into the blood supply near the left shoulder. From the right lymphatic duct lymph drains back into the bloodstream near the right shoulder.

Structure of the lymphatic system

The lymphatic system is like a stream of rivers and tributaries. Instead of water, all contain lymph, a salty, straw-coloured liquid like the fluid part of blood, but with less protein. The system's many tiny vessels join to form a few large ones. Largest of all is the thoracic duct which runs up the body in front of the spine. Another large vessel, the right lymphatic duct, runs through the right arm and shoulder. Bumpy swellings called lymph nodes occur in the neck and armpits, the groin and elsewhere. These contain white cells that absorb harmful substances such as bacteria.

The spleen

This organ plays a part in circulation and combatting infection. The spleen is a spongy, fist-sized, purplish object located just in front of the spine, below the diaphragm and left of and behind the stomach.

The spleen manufactures some of the blood formed in the body before birth. It contains cells that kill old or injured blood cells and destroy bacteria and parasites. It also produces antibodies and protein to attack viruses and other agents of infection.

Areas to work to help the lymphatic system

As the lymphatic system is distributed throughout the body, we do not need to isolate, on the feet, specific areas to help the lymphatic system, as we are in fact working out all these areas as we work on the entire body. However, in order to stimulate the thoracic duct which runs in front of the spine in the rib-cage area, by working out this area of the spine we would be assisting the stimulation of the lymphatic system.

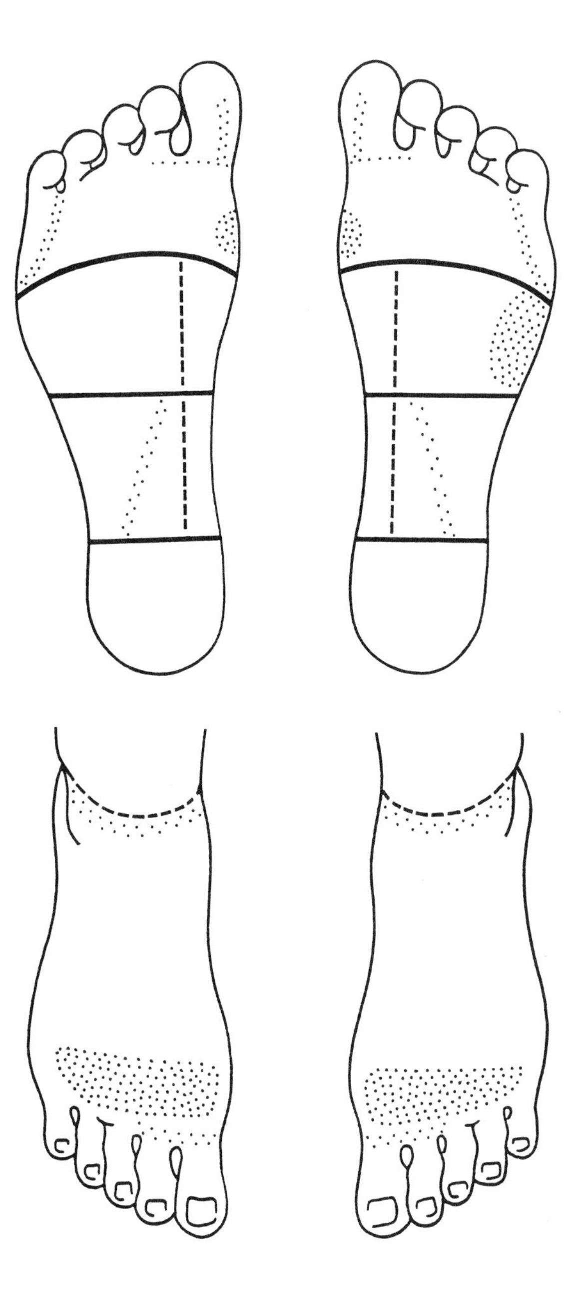

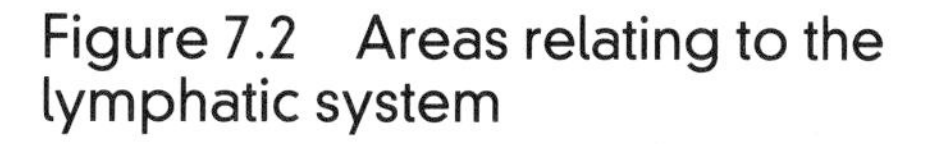

Figure 7.2 Areas relating to the lymphatic system

CHAPTER 8 The endocrine system

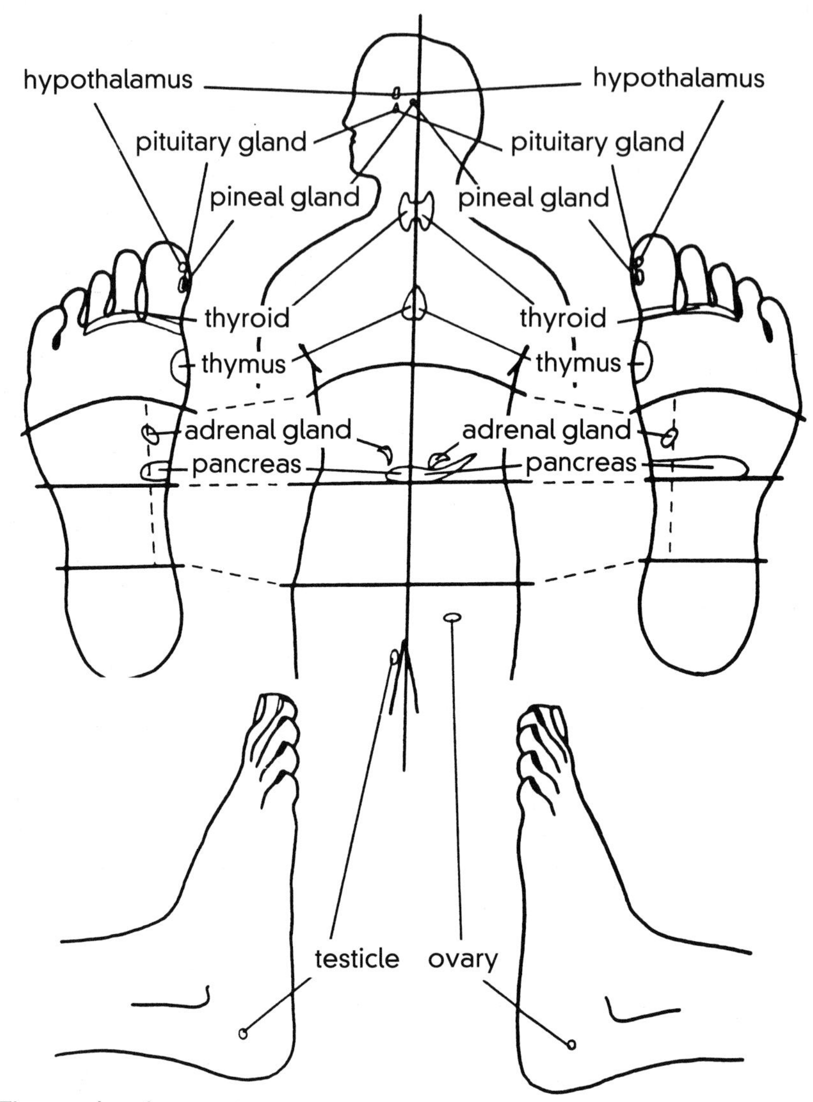

Figure 8.1 The endocrine system

The endocrine system consists of glands widely separated from one another with no direct anatomical links. They are commonly referred to as 'ductless glands' because the hormones they secrete pass directly into the bloodstream. A hormone is a chemical messenger which, having been formed in one organ or gland, is carried in the blood to another organ or tissue which is probably quite distant, where it influences activity, growth and nutrition. The internal environment of the body is controlled and regulated partly by the autonomic nervous system and partly by hormones.

The endocrine glands are as follows: the pituitary gland, the thyroid gland, four parathyroids, two adrenal glands, the Islets of Langerhans in the pancreas, one pineal gland or body, two ovaries in the female and two testes in the male.

The pituitary gland and hypothalamus

The pituitary gland and the hypothalamus act as one unit. Although the hypothalamus is classified as part of the brain and not as an endocrine gland, it has a direct controlling effect on the pituitary gland and an indirect effect on many others. The pituitary gland regulates the activity of most of the other endocrine glands. It is referred to as 'the master of the orchestra'. The gland lies between the eyes and behind the nose, and is protected by a very strong arch of bone called the sella turcica (or Turkish saddle). The pituitary gland has an anterior and posterior lobe. It controls many vital functions.

The pineal gland

The pineal gland is a small body situated in the fore-brain. It is connected to the brain by a short stalk containing nerves, many of which terminate in the hypothalamus. It is about 10mm long; it is reddish/brown in colour and surrounded by a capsule. Melatonin is the hormone secreted by the pineal gland. There is some direct association between the pineal gland and moods and behaviour patterns.

There is a link-up between the optic nerve and the pineal gland. Recent investigations in Greenland undertaken by a team of psychologists and psychiatrists studying the behaviour pattern of the Eskimo came to many interesting conclusions. In certain periods of the year, Eskimos have to live in semi-twilight. During this period, they frequently display strange behavioural patterns, such as manic-depressive states, hysterical and paranoid behaviour, and sometimes in extreme cases they lose the use of a limb or limbs. This is often referred to as 'hysterical paralysis'.

The psychologists came to the conclusion that these behaviour patterns resulted from the climatic conditions to which the Eskimos were subjected. As a daily routine, treatment was administered by ultra-violet ray into the area where the pineal gland is situated. The results were outstanding; most had treatment by this process for 20-minute sessions every day over the period of a month, and 90 per cent of sufferers regained their normal mental state. It is now felt that the pineal gland has some reflecting effect upon the brain which is transmitted via the optic nerve.

We all know the seasonal affective disorder commonly referred to as the SAD disease, which is quite common in England and many other cold countries. Many people find that during the autumn and winter months they tend to mimic the behavioural pattern of animals. They gain body weight, tend to become less active, sitting about more, and find that their mental activities become reduced. This behavioural change continues until spring, when the earth and life itself become vital again, light hours lengthen and the symptoms of seasonal affective disorder subside.

The main reason for these depressive symptoms is the lack of sunlight. Ultra-violet light seems to have a direct effect on mood, and in some way is absorbed via the eyes to the brain. Although most of us would agree that it is far better to look out on a sunny day than a grey, dismal one, you will now understand that it is not just an emotional response, but is in fact a basic physiological problem; we do need sun to keep us in good mental health.

This is probably the reason why the intake into psychiatric hospitals during the autumn and winter months is so high – a starvation of sunlight. It is therefore not surprising to find great sensitivity in the big toe area for those suffering from depression, anxiety and other stress-related conditions.

The thyroid gland

The thyroid gland, which also incorporates the parathyroids, stimulates growth and activity, and secretes the hormone thyroxine.

The thyroid is responsible for the metabolism of the body and for the extraction of iodine from the blood plasma, which has a significant influence on the mental health of individuals. A reduction of thyroxine can often cause severe neurotic tendencies. The hypothalamus in the brain secretes thyroid TRH (thyroid-releasing hormone).

The parathyroid glands lie embedded in the thyroid itself, and they contain a thick, sticky, semi-fluid structureless protein called colloid, in conjunction with which thyroid hormones are stored.

Between the follicles, there are cells called C cells and these secrete the hormone calcitonin.

The thymus

The thymus is a lymphatic gland which lies in front of the sternum and is large in young children. It supports the body against the invasion of severe disease in the very early years of life. It reduces in size until around puberty its function is minimal. The spleen then takes over the responsibility of protecting the immunity of the body.

Hormones

Growth hormone (GH) promotes growth of the skeleton, muscles, connective tissue and organs such as kidneys, liver, intestines, pancreas and adrenal glands.

Thyroid-stimulating hormone (TSH) stimulates growth and activity of the thyroid gland which secretes the hormone thyroxine. The function of the parathyroid is to secrete the hormone **parathormone**. Secretion is regulated by the blood level of calcium; when this falls, secretion is increased and vice versa. The main functions are to maintain the blood concentration of calcium within normal limits.

Adrenocorticotrophic hormone (ACTH) stimulates the flow of blood to the adrenal cortex, increases the concentration of cholesterol and steroids within the gland, and increases the output of steroid hormones, especially cortisol. ACTH levels are highest at about 8 a.m. and fall to their lowest about midnight, although high levels sometimes occur at midday and 6 p.m. This circadian rhythm is maintained throughout life; it is associated with the sleep pattern, and adjustment to changes take several days following (for example) shift work, or travel to a different time zone (jet lag).

Prolactin hormone has a direct effect on the breast immediately after childbirth. Suckling stimulates prolactin secretion and the result of a high prolactin hormone level in the blood is a factor in reducing the incident of conception during lactation.

Follicle-stimulating hormone (FSH) stimulates the development and ripening of the ovarian follicle. During its development the ovarian follicle secretes its own hormones. As the level of **oestrogen** increases in the blood, so FSH secretion is reduced. The **luteinizing hormone** promotes a final maturation of the ovarian follicle and ovulation. Its main function is to promote the formation of corpus luteum which secretes the second ovarian hormone, **progesterone**. As the level of progesterone in the blood increases, there is a gradual reduction in the production of the luteinizing hormone. The follicle-stimulating hormone in the male stimulates the epithelial tissue of the seminiferous tubule in the testes to produce spermatozoa. The luteinizing hormones stimulate the interstitial cells in the testes to secrete the hormone testosterone.

Oxytocin promotes contraction of uterine muscles and contraction of cells of the lactating breast, squeezing milk into the large ducts behind the nipple. In late pregnancy the uterus becomes very sensitive to oxytocin. The amount secreted will increase just before and during labour as well as by the suckling baby.

Anti-diuretic hormone (ADH) has two main functions. It increases the permeability to water of the distal, convoluting and collecting tubules of the nephron of the kidney. As a result, the re-absorption of water from the glomerular filtrate is increased, and the amount of ADH secreted is influenced by the osmotic pressure of the blood circulating. As the osmotic pressure rises, the secretion of the ADH increases and more water is re-absorbed. Conversely, when the osmotic pressure of the blood is low, the secretion of ADH is reduced, less water is re-absorbed and more urine is produced. The blood level is increased in dehydration and following haemorrhage. ADH stimulates contraction of smooth muscle, especially in the blood vessels, and abdominal organs, raising the blood pressure.

Islets of Langerhans (pancreas)

The cells which make up the Islets of Langerhans are found in clusters irregularly distributed throughout the substance of the pancreas. Unlike the pancreatic tissue, which reduces the digestive juice, there are no ducts leading from the clusters of islet cells. Their secretion passes directly into the pancreatic veins and circulates throughout the body. There are three main types of cell in the Islets of Langerhans: cells that secrete glucagon, cells that secrete insulin, and cells that secrete somatostatin. Insulin influences the level of glucose in the blood, and each balances the effects of the other. Glucagon tends to raise the blood – glucose level.

Conditions benefiting from reflexology

Stress and the endocrine system are closely linked. Therefore the conditions in which we are going to achieve the best results are tension states. Stress is in the main not destructive; in fact we all need to be stressed at times to be able to achieve anything. It is how the body copes with stress that is all important.

Some individuals thrive on stressful situations. In fact, they often go through life creating situations to activate stress levels in the body, because they perform better when in an emotionally high-powered state. It is when we are tense all the time that troubles in our health begin. In this situation, many people exhibit symptoms of illness, such as migraine, indigestion, colitis, asthma, back pain, to name but a few. We hold tension in our neck. How often have you said, 'He's a real pain in the neck,' when describing a person who creates in you bad, unsettled feelings? Our immune system becomes depressed when we are in a tense, anxious condition – too much nervous energy has been burnt up and so the general vitality of the body is affected, leaving us wide open for the onset of illness.

People who meditate or practise relaxation techniques regularly get the least disease of all – proof enough that relaxation and good feelings about oneself benefit the body. Racing through life like the speed of light, having little time 'to sit and stare', have a destructive effect.

The greatest benefit we can ever achieve with reflexology is relaxation of body, mind and spirit, the three essentials necessary for the healing process of the body to be set in motion.

Our adrenal glands are active glands which sit on top of each kidney and are very receptive to emotions and feelings.

The days when we all lived in caves and caught wild animals to survive have long past.

The release of adrenalin during these times was enormous, as either the wild animals ate us up and that was the end of that, or we killed the beasts and had food for our family for some time.

What actually happens when we are tense, anxious or even frightened? If we relate to the caveman, he stalked his prey, with adrenalin coursing though his veins. He stealthily walked through the jungle, nerves quivering at any movement or sound, his pupils dilated to enable him to see better, his blood was already thickening in his veins so that it would be able to clot faster if he was wounded. His bronchial tubes dilated to enable him to take in more oxygen, his heart was already beating faster to distribute the oxygen around his body, preparing him to 'run for his life'. He probably had a great desire to urinate or have a bowel movement. (I am sure you have often felt the urgent desire to urinate frequently or open your bowels when confronting a situation in your life which made you fearful, such as taking an examination, or confronting an audience to make an after-dinner speech.) That anxiety state is a remnant left from the most primitive forms of life when, to enable you to 'run for your life', you needed to be as weightless as possible!

Glucose and fats were being released from his liver. He needed these elements to give him extra energy and power. Every muscle in his body was vibrating, even his hearing was more acute as he 'listened and watched'.

The wild boar came into view and he ran with his mallet positioned above his head and attacked it. All the energy in his body was stimulated to its peak performance by those two little caps that sit on top of the kidneys – the adrenal glands.

Having killed his prey he tied a rope around the carcass and dragged it back to his cave. The energy used to kill his prey was enormous, and after this experience he slept for many hours to recover from the emotional and physical event. This is exactly how the body was meant to perform.

However, today we live in a totally different stress-related world. We confront stressful situations all the time, because we are living in a fast-changing world, with changes that we can hardly keep up with. If you look back fifty years and list the changes that have occurred in that period, it is incredible. We don't have the anxiety of the wild boar, but we could have a patronising, difficult boss to contend with who releases in us all sorts of emotions, from anger to utter despair. We live in fear of redundancy, we fight through traffic jams, and worry about the future of our children in a world packed with so much violence.

Our bodies produce the same symptoms and hormones when we experience situations that give rise to anxiety, fear and tension. The big problem is that we never have the opportunity to run for our life or burn off, by extreme physical exercise, the excess of adrenalin in our veins. So our body has the excess of fats, glucose and adrenalin in our veins which just permeate our entire circulatory system clogging up our arteries and causing all the cardio-vascular diseases which are paramount today.

We need more exercise and relaxation, a balance of both. What better way to achieve total relaxation than reflexology? The type of exercise you decide must be up to you.

There is no case history in particular that stands out in my mind which relates to the endocrine system.

Generally speaking, reflexology is of great benefit in the relief of menstrual and menopausal discomforts, and it has proved to be of value in helping infertility. I had two patients who were unable to conceive due to infrequent ovulation. Within three months both patients conceived and proclaimed the true virtues of reflexology. Many of my practitioners throughout the country have had similar results with their patients.

Practical procedures for working the endocrine system

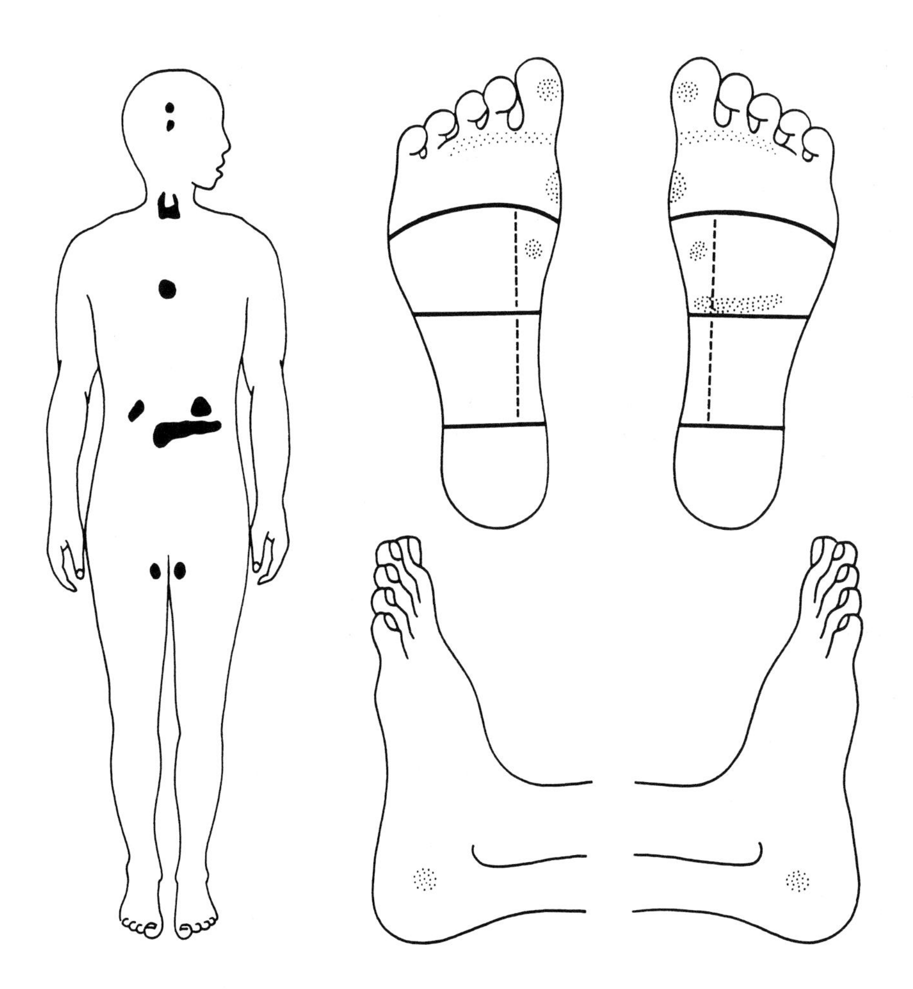

Figure 8.2 Areas relating to the endocrine system

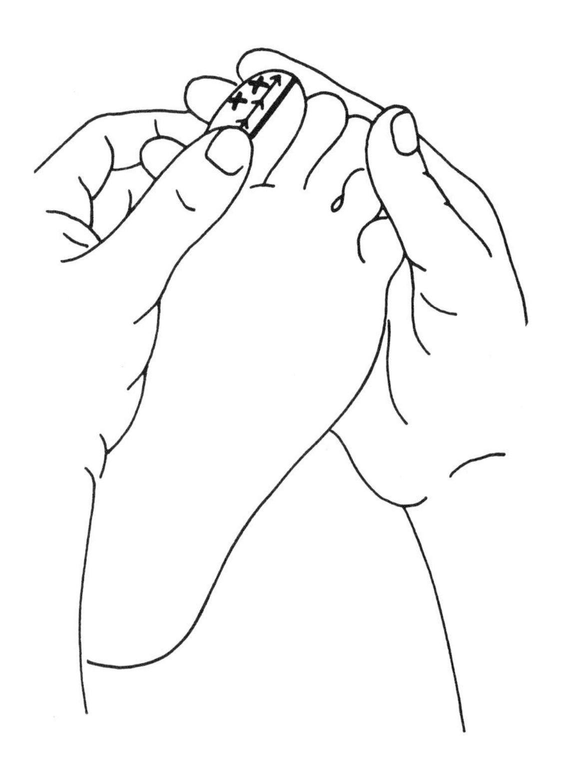

Figure 8.3 The pituitary gland and hypothalamus and the pineal gland (left foot), plantar view, zone 1, medial.
Supporting the left foot at the top with your right hand and using the left thumb, work two or three times up the big toe (medial side only).

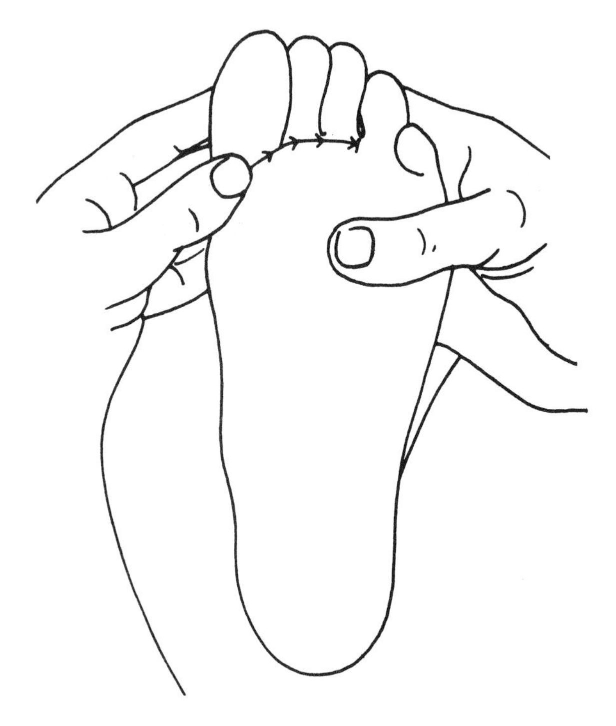

Figure 8.4 The thyroid/neck area (left foot), plantar view, zones 1 2 3, medial to lateral.
Supporting the left foot at the top with your right hand and using the left thumb, work two or three times across this area.

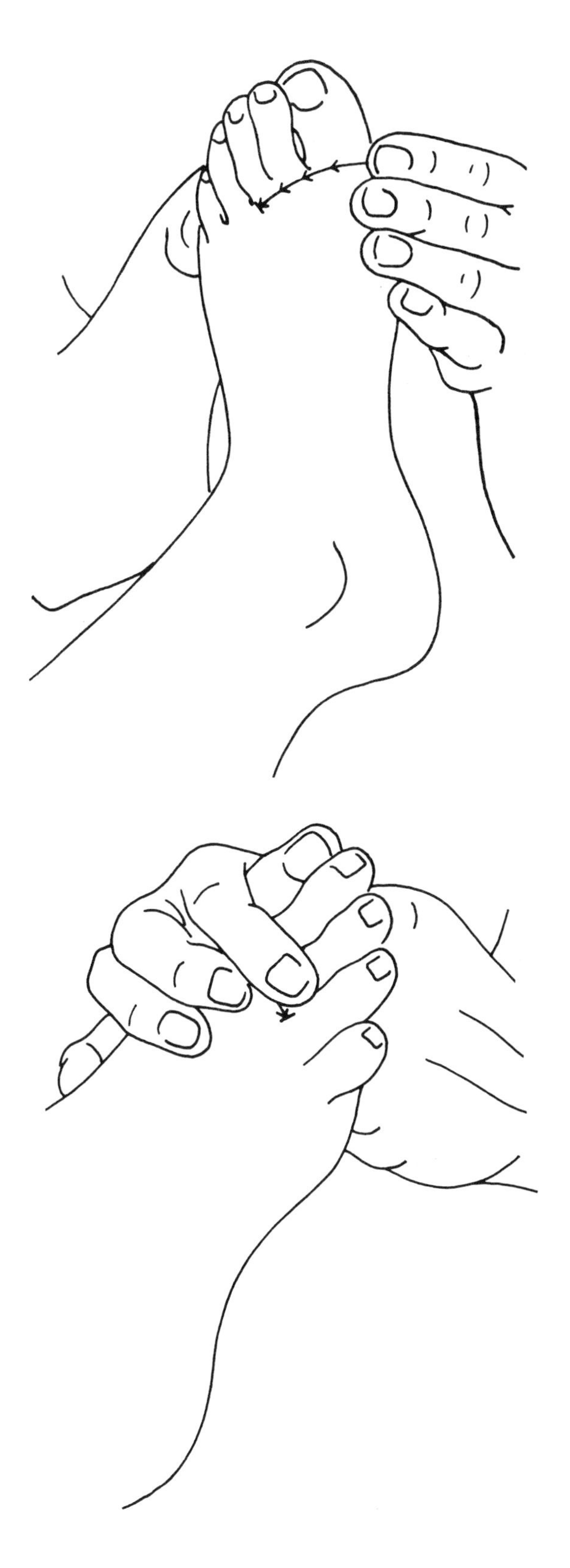

Figure 8.5 The thyroid/neck area (left foot), dorsal view, top support, zones 1 2 3, medial to lateral.
Supporting the left foot with your right fist and using the left index finger, work two or three times across this line.

Figure 8.6 The thyroid/neck area (right foot), dorsal view, zones 1 2 3.
Work the thyroid/neck area ending at the third toe.

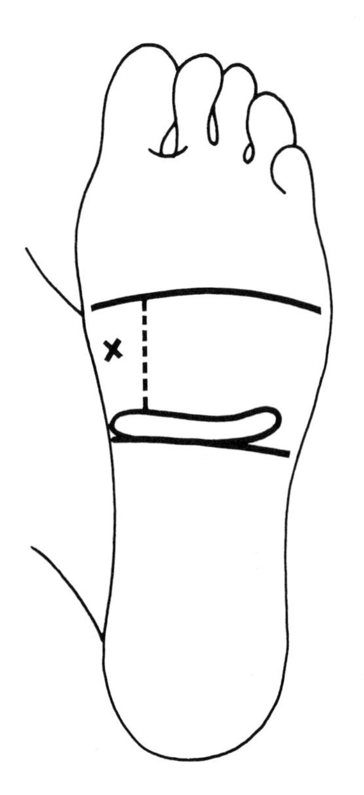

Figure 8.7 The adrenal gland and pancreas (left foot), plantar view.
The practical procedures for working these areas were covered in the digestive system (see Figures 4.11 and 4.12). However, be aware of exactly where these reflexes are to be found in the feet, noting that the pancreas is on the left foot only.

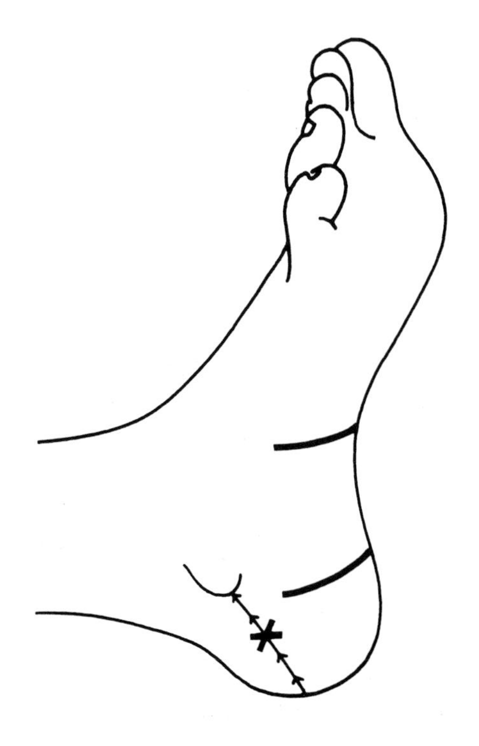

Figure 8.8 The ovary/testes (right foot), lateral view.
The practical procedures for working this area are to be found in the reproductive system (see Figure 13.7). The 'X' identifies the exact position for the ovary/testes.

CHAPTER 9 The solar plexus

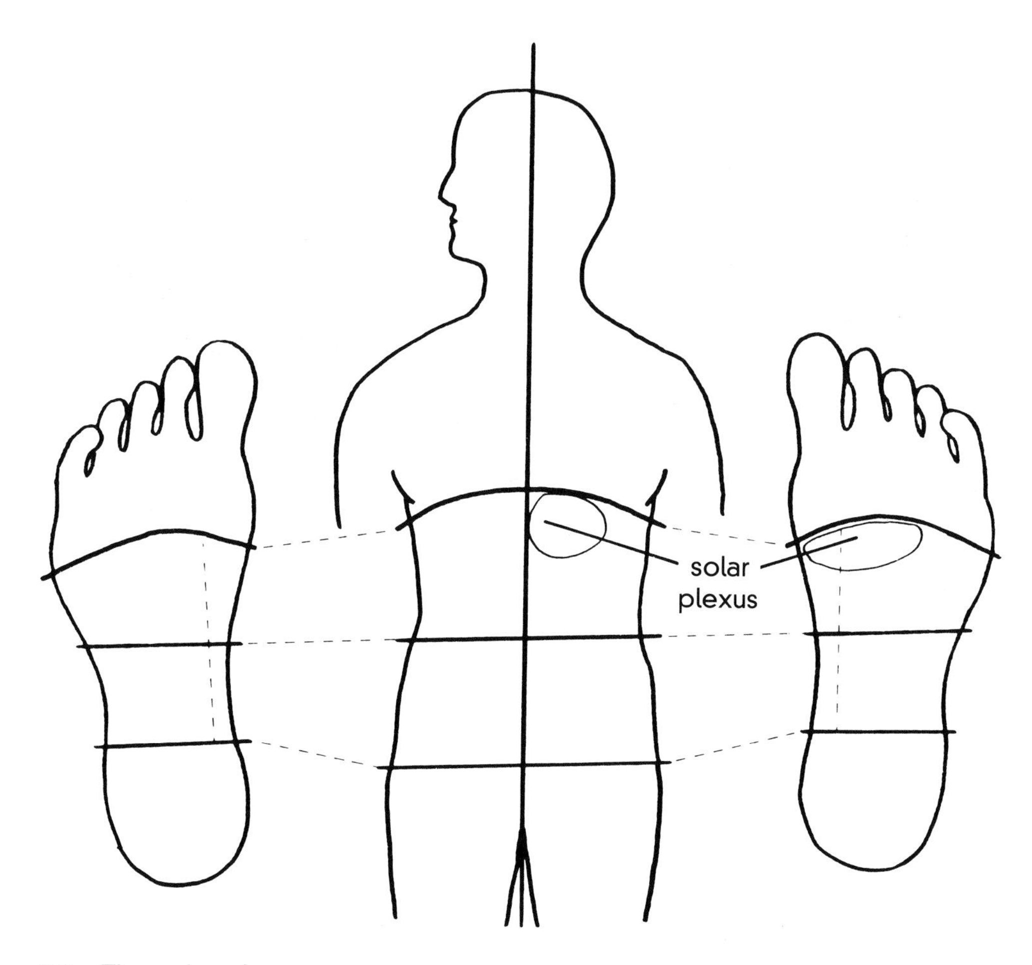

Figure 9.1 The solar plexus

The solar plexus is a network of nerves which lies behind the stomach wall. 'Solar' is from the word 'sun', and 'plexus', 'a grouping together of nerves'.

When we work on the solar plexus – which we will do automatically as we work on the digestive system on the left side of the body – we will be making contact with this area frequently. This is all to the good, as it does create a feeling of well-being and has a relaxing effect upon the body.

Generally, it is quite usual to pick up a lot of sensitivity in this area when treating patients who are under a lot of emotional 'strains and pains'.

The solar plexus sends out signals in the form of 'butterflies in the stomach' when you are feeling particularly nervous. Maybe there is an impending interview, or you have received sad or exciting news about a friend. These strange, vibratory signals are all being sent out by our good friend 'the solar plexus'.

Areas to work to help the solar plexus

It is not necessary to work out the area to the solar plexus separately as it lies on the left foot behind the stomach area, just below the diaphragm line, and so it is worked out automatically as one treats the stomach area. However, it is a very good identification of extreme stress in a patient and in many instances pressure applied to this area can result in extreme sensitivity when working with patients who are perhaps going through a traumatic period of their lives and are in an anxious condition. It is therefore a 'barometer to your emotional health'.

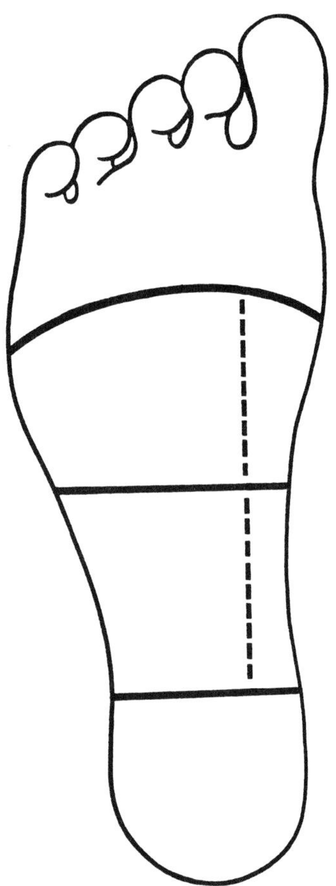

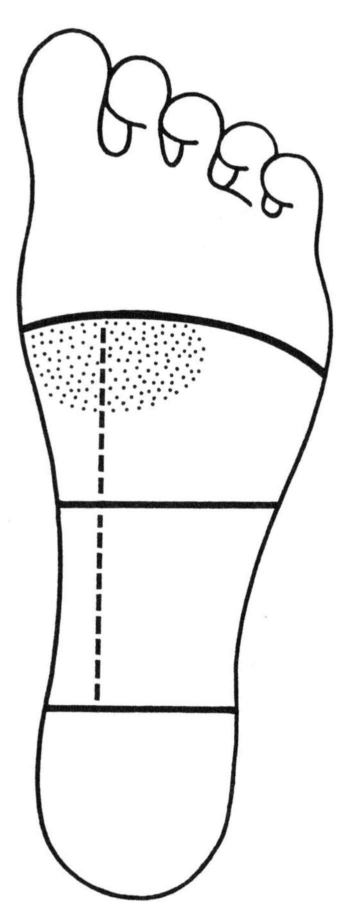

Figure 9.2 Areas relating to the solar plexus

FOOT CHART

FOOT CHART

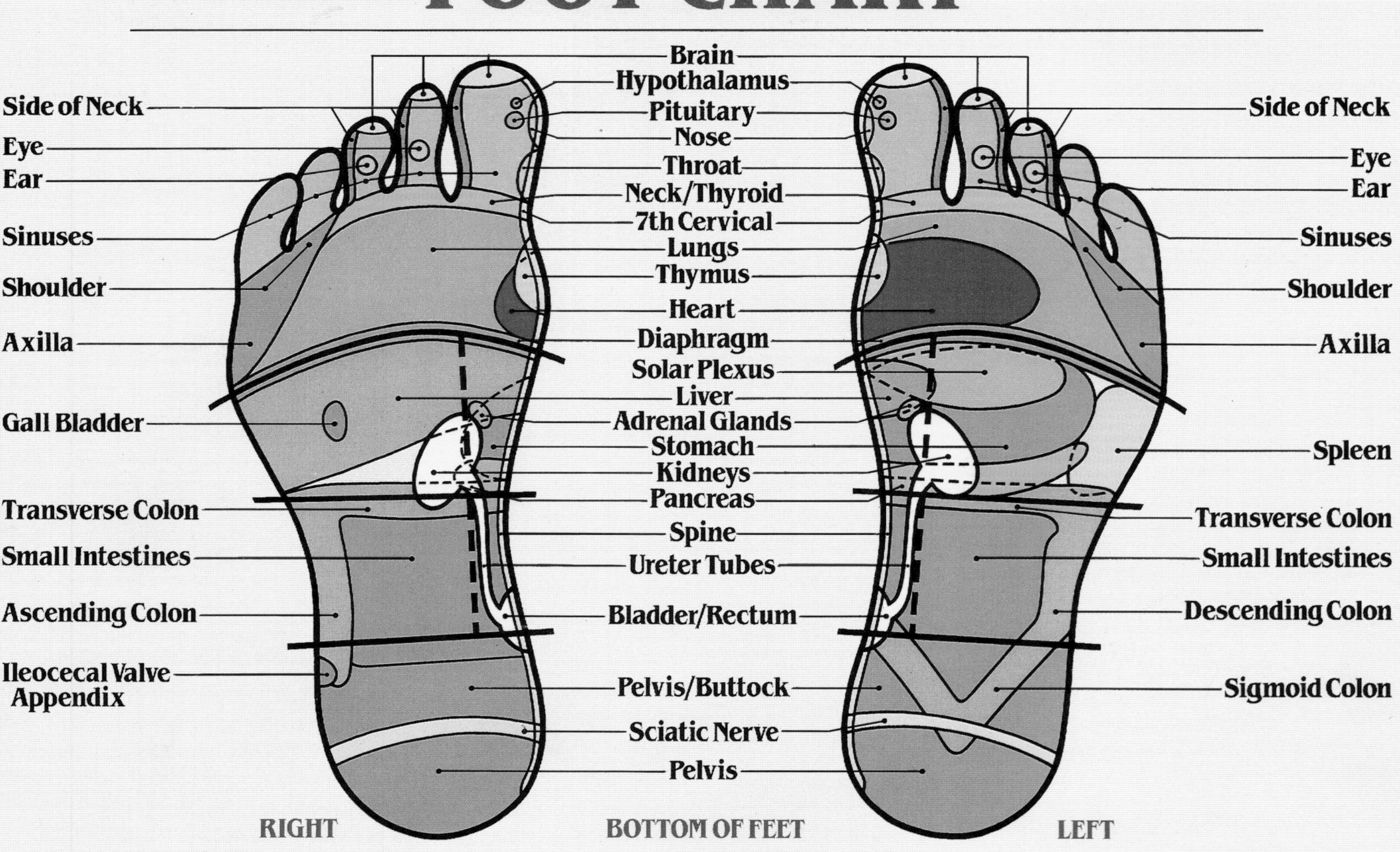

Side of Neck
Eye
Ear
Sinuses
Shoulder
Axilla
Gall Bladder
Transverse Colon
Small Intestines
Ascending Colon
Ileocecal Valve
Appendix
Brain
Hypothalamus
Pituitary
Nose
Throat
Neck/Thyroid
7th Cervical
Lungs
Thymus
Heart
Diaphragm
Solar Plexus
Liver
Adrenal Glands
Stomach
Kidneys
Pancreas
Spine
Ureter Tubes
Bladder/Rectum
Pelvis/Buttock
Sciatic Nerve
Pelvis
Side of Neck
Eye
Ear
Sinuses
Shoulder
Axilla
Spleen
Transverse Colon
Small Intestines
Descending Colon
Sigmoid Colon
RIGHT
BOTTOM OF FEET
LEFT

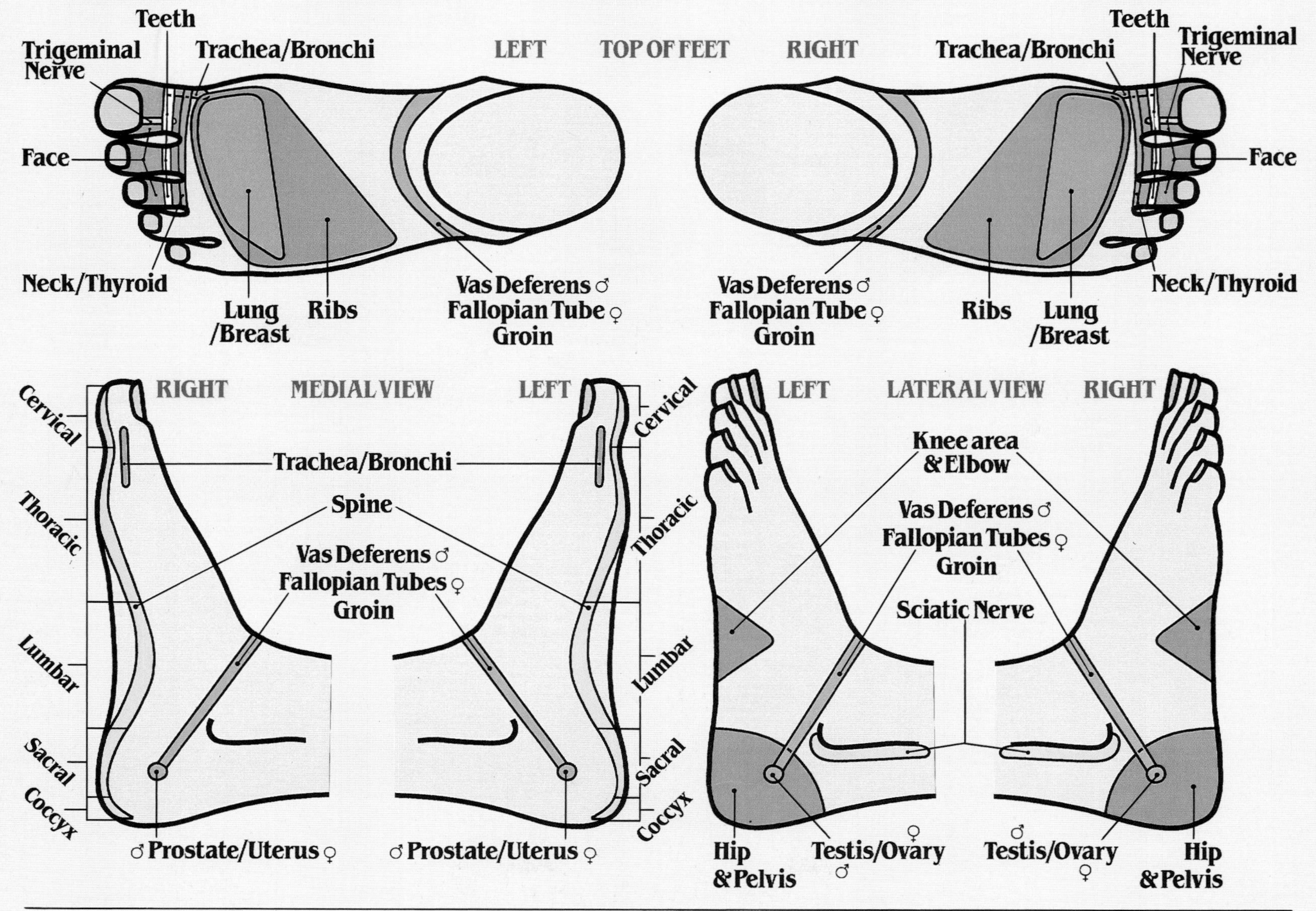
LEFT
TOP OF FEET
RIGHT
Teeth
Trigeminal Nerve
Trachea/Bronchi
Face
Neck/Thyroid
Lung /Breast
Ribs
Vas Deferens ♂
Fallopian Tube ♀
Groin
Teeth
Trigeminal Nerve
Trachea/Bronchi
Face
Neck/Thyroid
Ribs
Lung /Breast
Vas Deferens ♂
Fallopian Tube ♀
Groin
RIGHT
MEDIAL VIEW
LEFT
Cervical
Thoracic
Lumbar
Sacral
Coccyx
Trachea/Bronchi
Spine
Vas Deferens ♂
Fallopian Tubes ♀
Groin
♂ Prostate/Uterus ♀
♂ Prostate/Uterus ♀
Cervical
Thoracic
Lumbar
Sacral
Coccyx
LEFT
LATERAL VIEW
RIGHT
Knee area & Elbow
Vas Deferens ♂
Fallopian Tubes ♀
Groin
Sciatic Nerve
Hip & Pelvis
Testis/Ovary ♀ ♂
Testis/Ovary ♂ ♀
Hip & Pelvis

CHAPTER 10 The central nervous system, eye, ear, nose, throat, sinuses and face

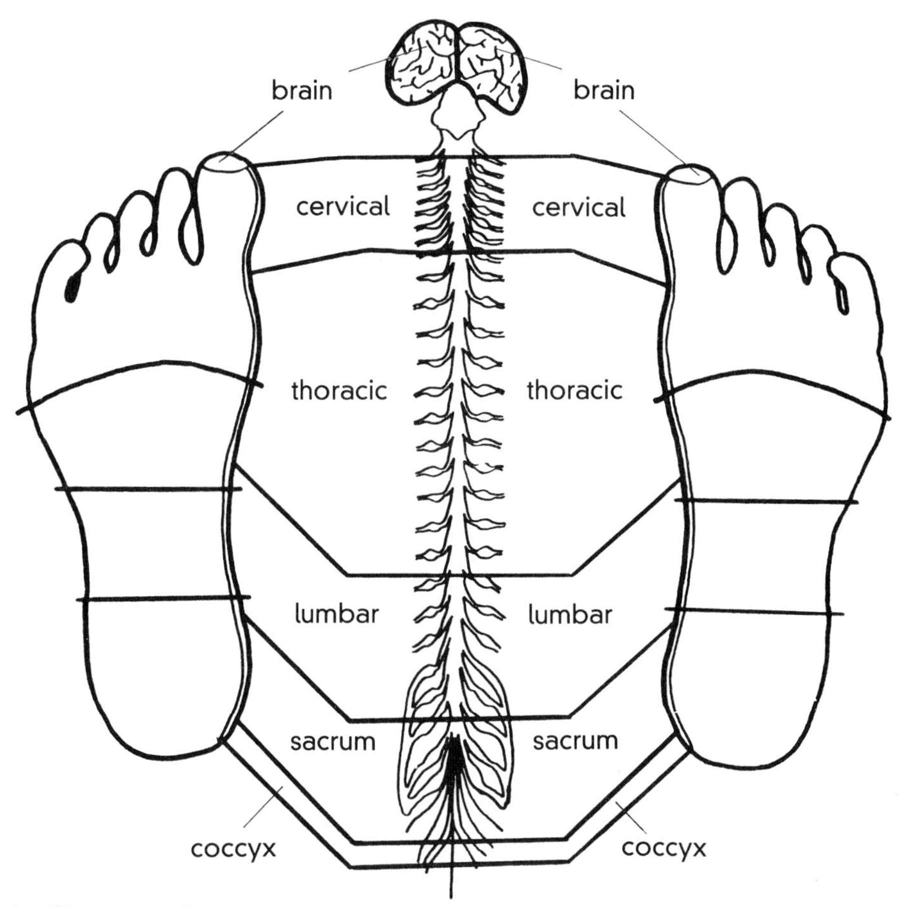

Figure 10.1 The central nervous system

The brain and spinal cord comprise the central nervous system. The brain's billions of nerve cells (neurones) control consciousness, emotions, thought, movement and unconscious body functions.

Brain structure

The brain looks like a giant wrinkled walnut crammed inside the skull. It is encased by two membranes, or meninges, which contain the cerebrospinal fluid, cushioning it against damage. Its main parts are the cerebrum, the cerebellum and the brain stem. The cerebrum takes up about seven-tenths of the nervous system. It comprises a right cerebral hemisphere and a left cerebral hemisphere, connected deep down by a mass of linking fibres. The cerebrum's deeply wrinkled cortex (the surface layer) contains grey matter (nerve

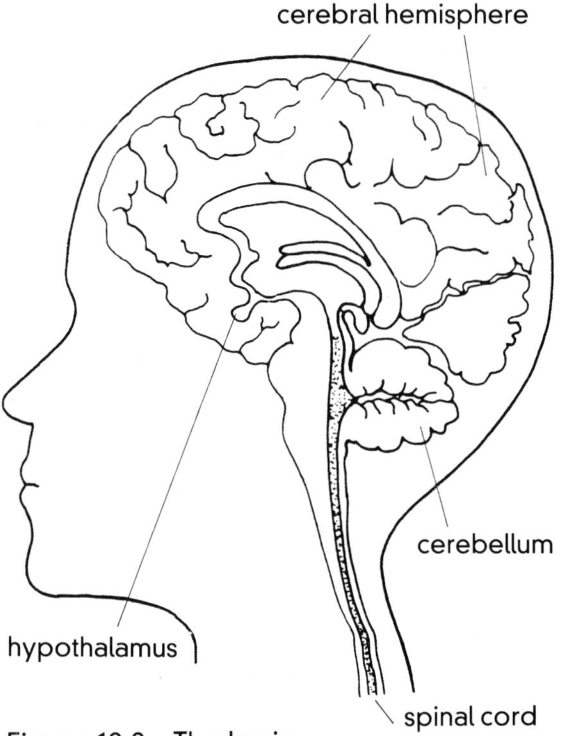

Figure 10.2 The brain

cells) over-lying white matter (nerve trunks). Certain cerebral areas deal with special functions: the motor cortex with voluntary movement; the sensory cortex with bodily sensations; the frontal lobe with personality; the occipital lobe with control of sight and the centre of the brain is the hearing and speech centre.

Below the mass of fibres linking the cerebral hemispheres lie the hypothalamus and other control co-ordination and relay centres. Some control the emotions and behaviour.

The cerebellum is the second largest region of the brain and it projects below the back of the cerebrum. This structure deals with balance and co-ordination of complex movements of the body. The brain stem is a stalk of nerve fibres, a nucleus that joins the spinal cord to the cerebellum and the cerebrum. Brain stem centres automatically control activities like breathing, heart beat and digestion.

Neurones

A neurone consists of a rounded cell body from which project long insulating fibres, the axon and branching dendrites.

Neurones are nerve cells. A neurone network forms the nervous system. Sensory neurones send signals from nerve endings in the eye, ear, skin and so on to the brain. Motor neurones send signals from the brain and spinal cord to muscles. Inter neurones provide intervening links.

A sensory neurone and motor neurone each have three main parts, a rounded cell body, a long, narrow insulated axon and branching dendrites. Electrical impulses flow along the axon and dendrites, and chemical messengers jump the gaps (synapse) between one neurone and another. Impulses may be afferent to or efferent from the nerve cell.

The spinal cord

This soft, curved cylinder of nerve fibre is about 45.7cm long and runs from the brain through the vertebral canal. From the spinal cord thirty-one pairs of nerves branch out into the body. These spinal nerves, plus twelve pairs of cranial nerves rooted in the brain, form the so-called peripheral nervous system.

The peripheral nervous system

The peripheral nerves help form the somatic and autonomic nervous system. The somatic system involves sensory nerves which send signals from sense organs to the central nervous system and motor nerves which send signals from the central nervous system to muscles under voluntary control.

The **autonomic nervous system** is composed of the sympathetic and parasympathetic systems, and produce actions that balance one another. Probably directed by the hypothalamus in the brain, they handle activities outside conscious control.

The **sympathetic nervous system** sends blood to the brain, heart, lungs, and so on preparing us for bodily exertion. Nerves from the spinal cord, thoracic and lumbar regions pass through nerve knots (ganglia) to act on different organs.

The **parasympathetic nervous system** dominates the sympathetic nervous system when we are at rest. It reduces much of the activity that the system triggers, reducing the heart rate but sending blood to the intestines and increasing output of digestive juices.

Nerves from the brain stem and spinal cord's central region act on different organs, such as ears.

The ears

Ears contain structures that enable us to hear and keep our balance. The human ear is sensitive to sounds ranging in loudness from 10 to 140 decibels (10 million million times as loud as 10), and ranging in pitch from 20 to a high 20,000 hertz cycles per second.

The distance between the ears helps the brain to locate the direction of the sound and its source. The structure of the ears is as follows. Each ear comprises three parts: the outer ear, the middle ear and the inner ear. The outer ear consists of a cartilage flap, the pinna, and the meatus or ear canal.

The middle ear has an ear-drum leading to three tiny bones or ossicles, the mallus (the hammer), incus (anvil) and stapes (stirrup). The Eustachian tube opens into the back of the throat and keeps the middle ear air pressure the same as that outside.

The inner ear contains a coiled, fluid-filled tube, a cochlea, with a so-called oval window and round window containing the organ of Corti with nerve cells connected to the auditory nerve. The organ of balance comprises three fluid filled semi-circular canals (U-shaped tubes) containing hairs sensitive to movement and cells sensing bodily position.

How hearing works

The pinna funnels send waves through the ear canal, where they vibrate the ear-drum. The ossicles amplify this vibration and transmit it by the oval window to the fluid in the cochlea. Here, cells in the organ of Corti interpret vibrations as nerve impulses carried by the auditory nerve to the brain. Meanwhile, vibrations leave the cochlea through the round window.

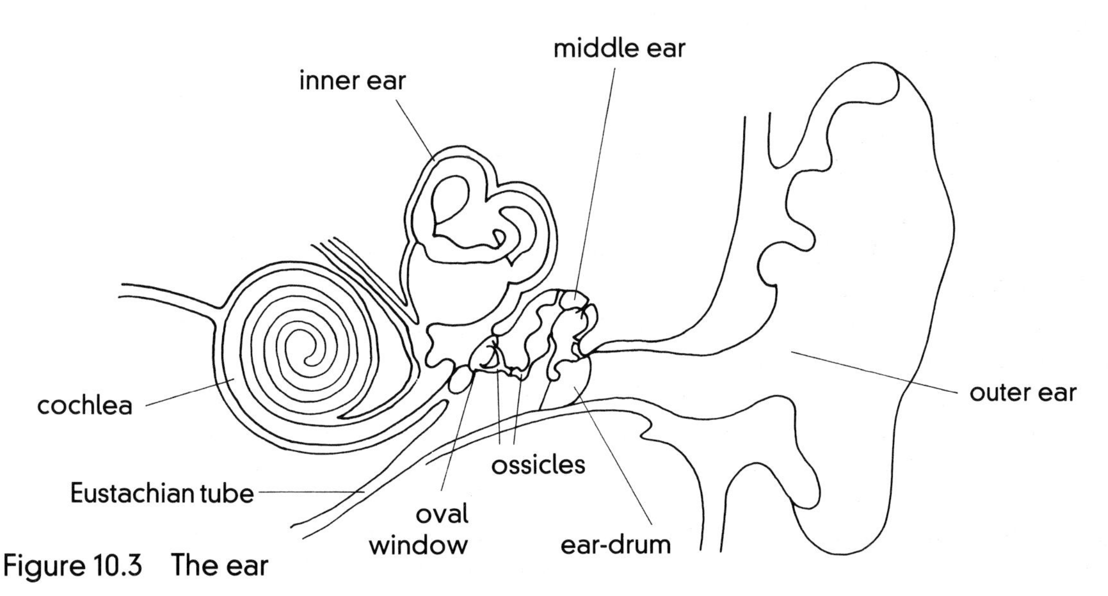

Figure 10.3 The ear

The eyes

We see the world around us by sensing the light that objects give off or reflect. Eyes look like two balls of jelly each about 2.5cm across, set in and protected by sockets called orbits in the skull on each side of the nose. The optic nerve at the rear of each eye sends messages from the eyeball to the visual cortex of the brain. Overlapping fields of vision help depth perception. Eyelids and eyelashes protect eyes from dust and injury.

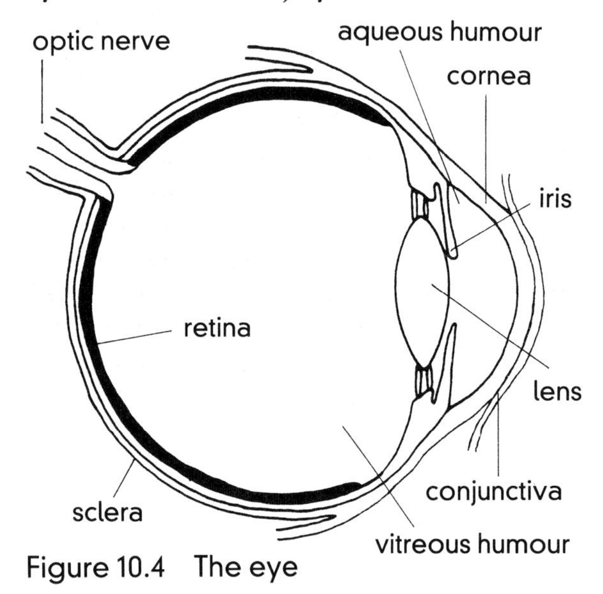

Figure 10.4 The eye

Parts of the eye

The sclera, or white, forms the outer layer of the eyeball. At the front of the eye the transparent cornea replaces the sclera. The cornea is covered by a thin protective membrane called the conjunctiva, which is lubricated by salty fluid secreted by the lacrimal gland on the inside of the upper eyelid.

Behind the cornea lies the anterior chamber of the eye, containing the watery fluid, aqueous humour. This is separated from the posterior chamber by the lens. The posterior chamber contains vitreous humour, a much firmer jelly giving the eyeball its firmness. In front of the lens is a circular muscle, the iris, which gives the eye its colour. Light is admitted through the central black hole, or pupil, to the back of the eye through the lens to focus on the retina. The light is focused as it passes through the cornea and aqueous humour.

Inside the eye, light rays from an object are bent by the cornea, lens, aqueous humour and vitreous humour so that the rays come to focus on the retina. The focused image is upside down, but the brain sees it the right way up. Light rays from a distant object are bent relatively slightly inside the eye. Its lens has slightly curved sides.

The sense of smell

Cells sensitive to smell occur in the olfactory nerves. They have their origins in special cells in the mucus membrane of the roof of the nose above the superior nasal passage. On each side of the nasal septum nerve fibres from the cells pass through the nasal area.

The sense of smell in human beings is generally less acute than in other animals. All odorous materials give off chemical particles which are carried into the nose with the inhaled air and stimulate nerve cells of the olfactory region when dissolved in mucus.

When an individual is continuously exposed to an odour, perception of the odour quickly decreases and eventually ceases.

Air entering the nose is heated and convection currents carry eddies of inspired air from the main stream to the roof of the nose. 'Sniffing' concentrates more particles more quickly to the roof of the nose. This increases the number of special cells stimulated and thus the perception of the smell. The sense of smell may affect the appetite. If the odours are pleasant the appetite may improve and vice versa.

Inflammation of the nasal mucosa prevents odorous substances from reaching the olfactory area of the nose causing loss of the sense of smell. The usual cause is the common cold.

How reflexology can help

The types of conditions reflexologists are able to help relieve in connection with the nervous system are: multiple sclerosis; Parkinson's disease; eye and ear conditions, particularly tinnitus; constant ear, nose and throat conditions in children; tired, strained eyes and conjunctivitis.

Many people going through an extremely stressful situation in their lives find that their eyesight deteriorates rapidly. This is caused by tension and by relieving the stress and tension with reflexology their eyesight quickly returns to its normal state.

Sinus conditions frequently affect the areas of taste and smell, and also cause extreme congestion in the nasal cavities, which in turn causes pressure, pain and infection in the facial areas. Sinusitis is often caused by an infection which comes about after a heavy cold, leaving you with catarrh. Alternatively, it can be complicated by an episode of hay fever, which causes irritation and infection to the linings of the nose and throat. These conditions can be easily relieved by reflexology.

Unfortunately, one of the most common conditions affecting the functions of the brain is a stroke or cerebral vascular accident. A stroke has nothing to do with a heart atack. It is in fact an eruption of a weakened blood vessel in the brain, and is frequently caused by a history of high blood pressure. Eventually the increased pressure on the artery wall causes a weakening, just like a worn area in a car tyre, which eventually bulges out and causes a break in its structure. When this 'accident' occurs, blood seeps into the brain area causing pressure on vital brain cells, frequently causing paralysis of the use of one side of the body, and very often the patient will lose the ability to speak, if the speech centre is affected. Providing reflexology can be carried out as soon after the episode as possible, excellent results are obtainable. I believe that even though the stroke may cause a lot of brain damage, there is usually some small nerve impulse remaining to be stimulated, which in turn will help the functions of the brain to become restored.

Practical procedures for working the central nervous system, eye, ear, nose, throat, sinuses and face

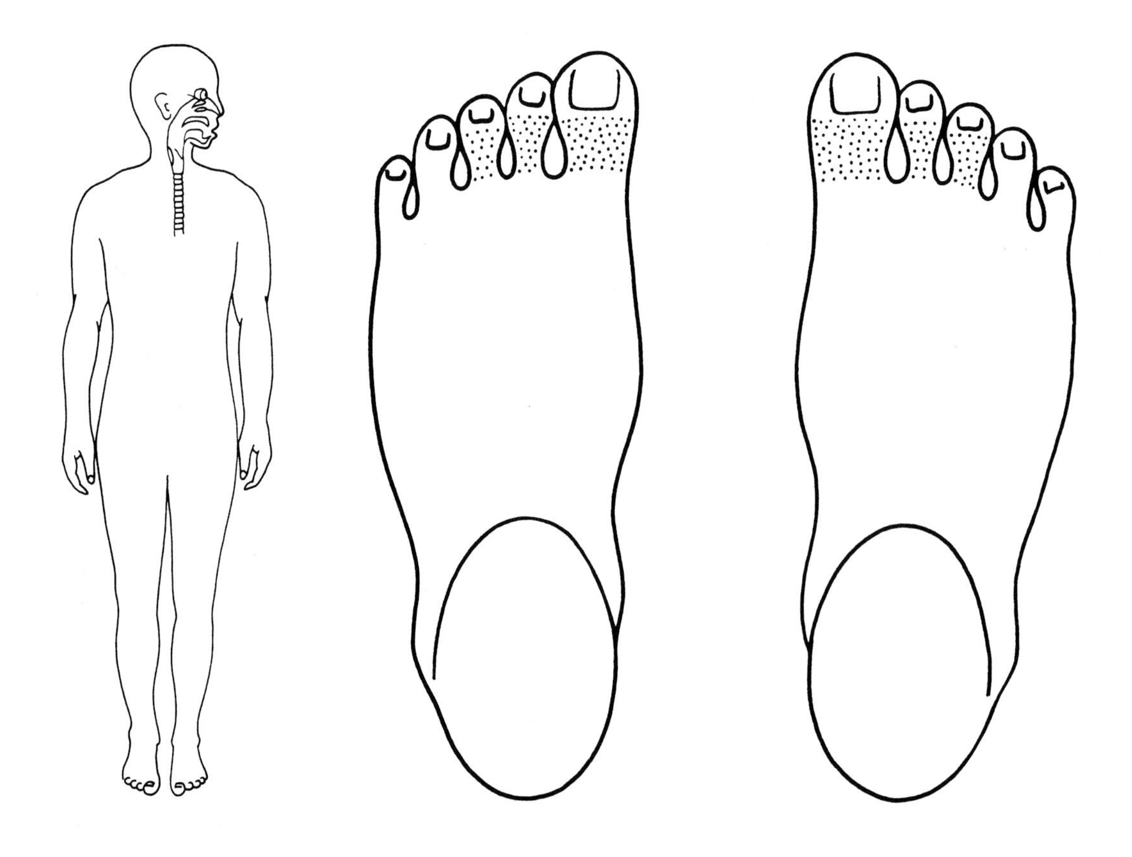

Figure 10.5 Areas relating to the face

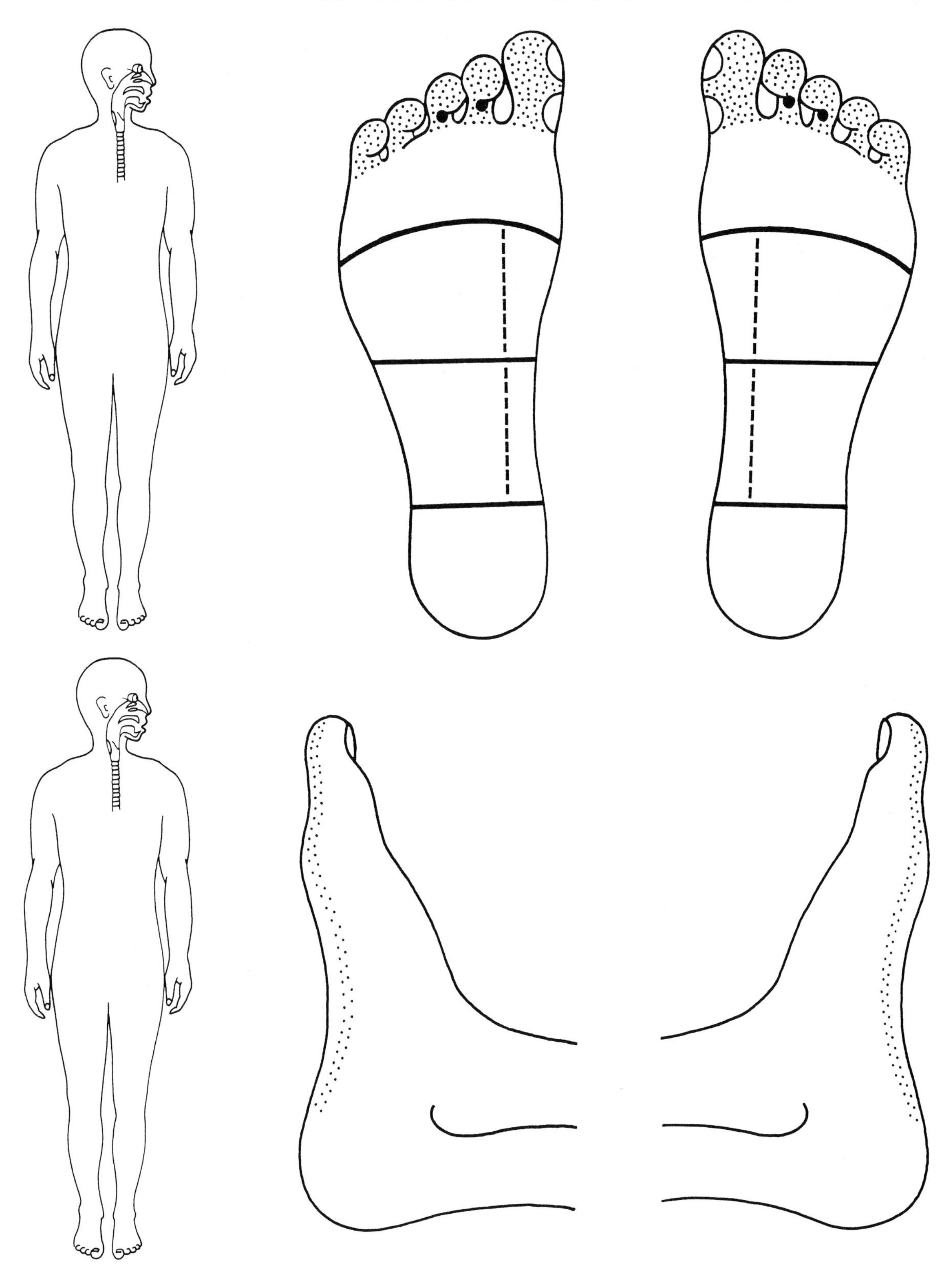

Figure 10.6 Areas relating to the eye, ear, nose, throat and sinuses

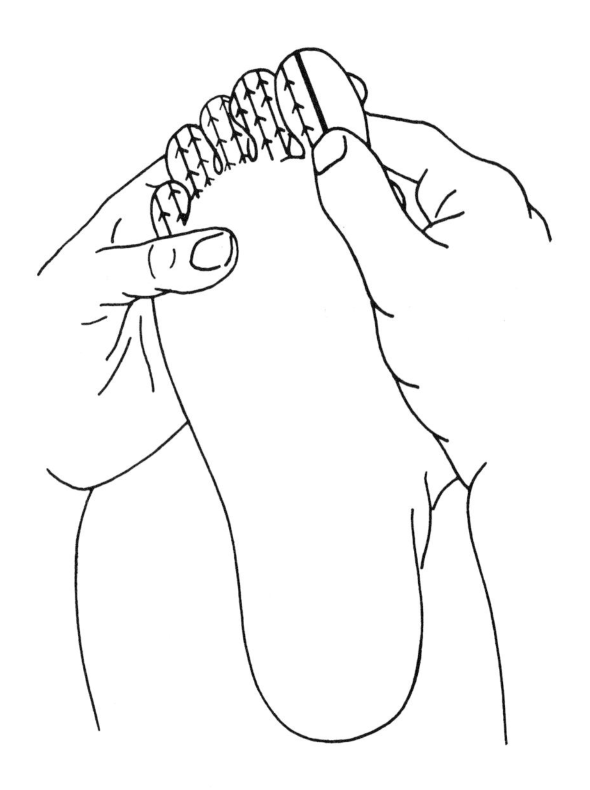

Figure 10.7 The sinus areas (right foot), plantar view, top support, zones 1 2 3 4 5, medial to lateral.
Supporting the right foot with your left hand, work out the areas identified with the right thumb.

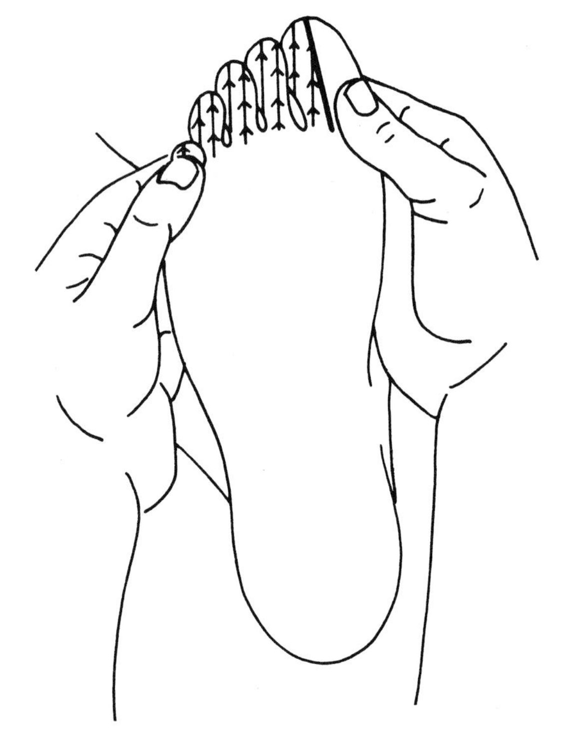

Figure 10.8 The sinus areas (right foot), plantar view, top support, zones 1 2 3 4 5, lateral to medial.
Supporting the right foot with your right hand, work with the left thumb.

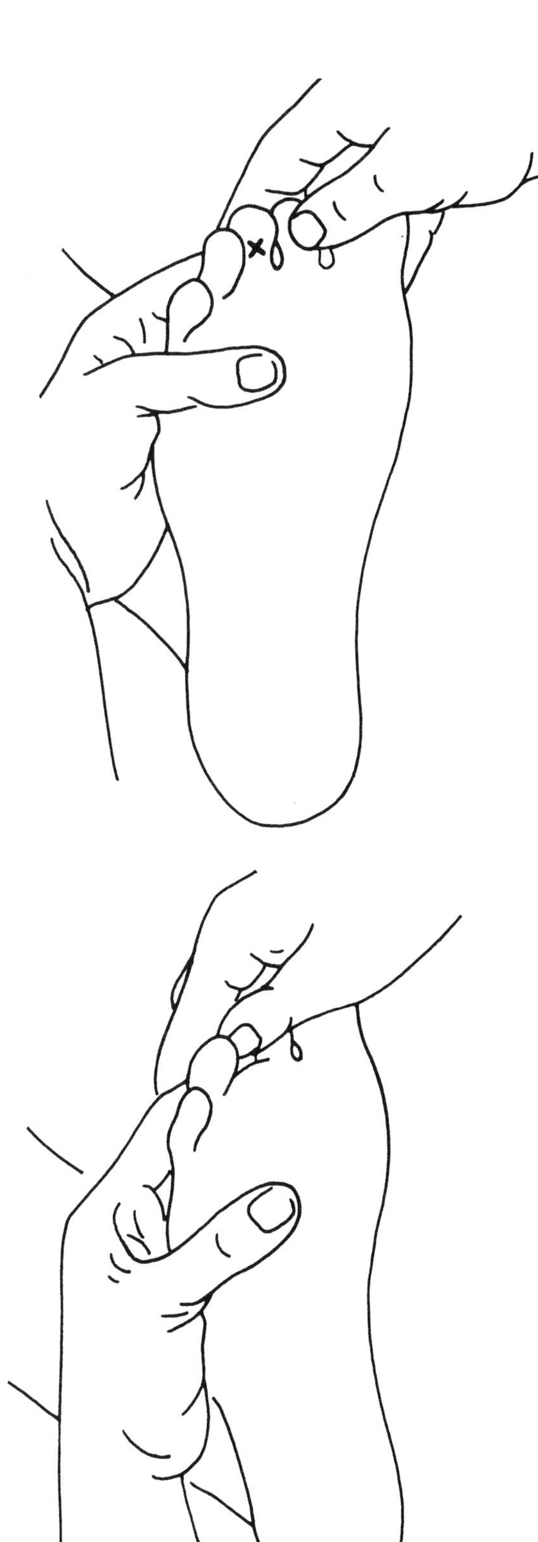

Figure 10.9 The eye (right foot), plantar view, top support, zone 2.
Supporting the right foot with your left hand, use a gentle rotating movement with the right thumb.

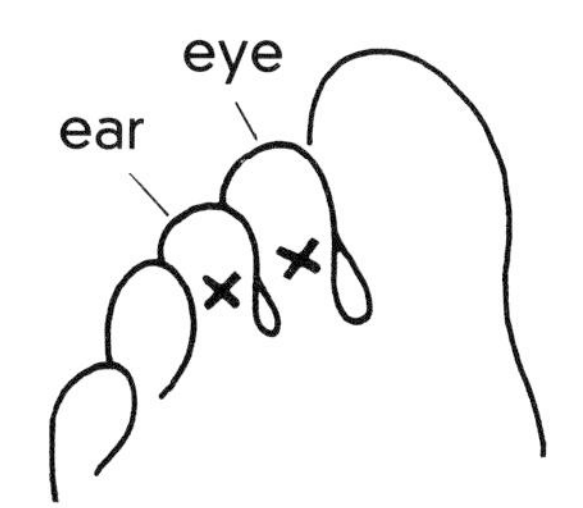

Figure 10.10 The ear (right foot), top support, zone 3.
Supporting the right foot with your left hand, use a gentle rotating movement with the right thumb.

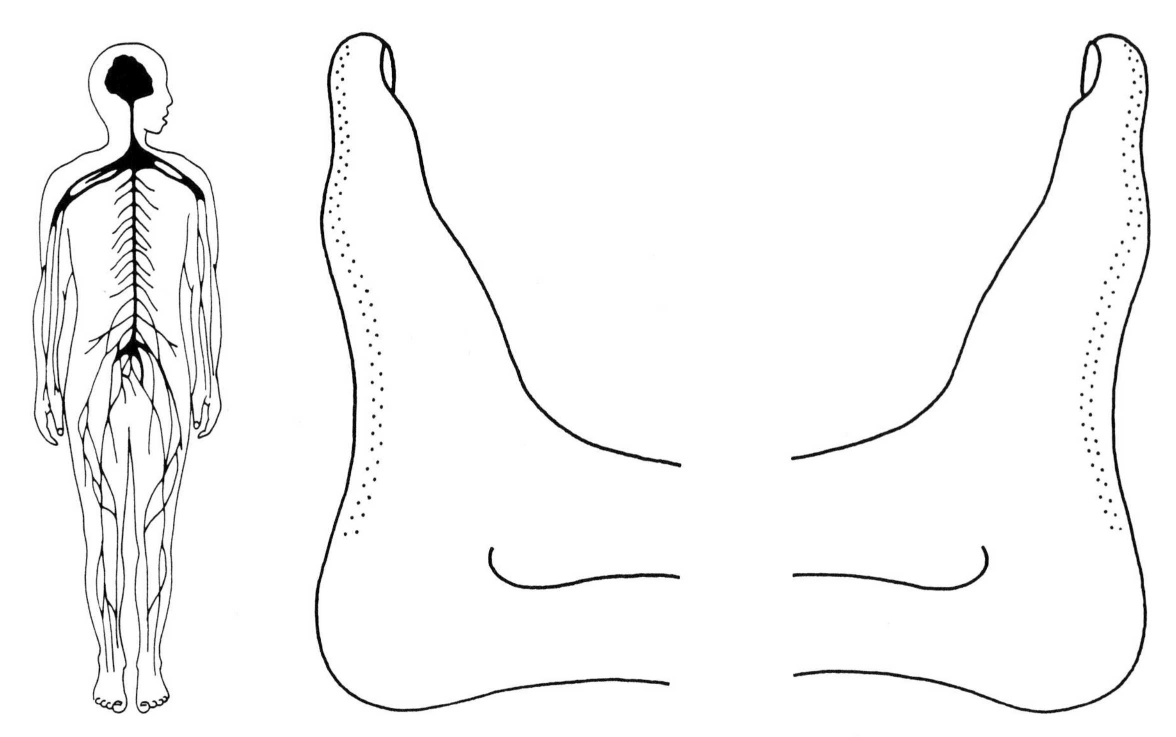

Figure 10.11 Areas relating to the central nervous system

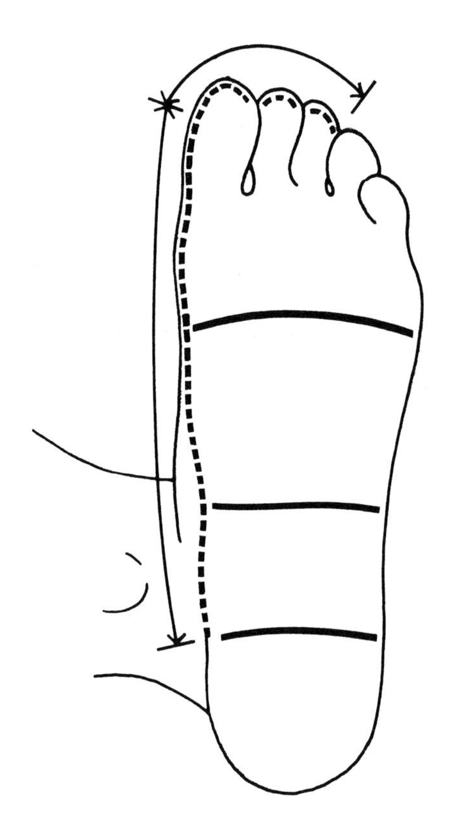

Figure 10.12 The areas of the spinal cord and brain (left foot).

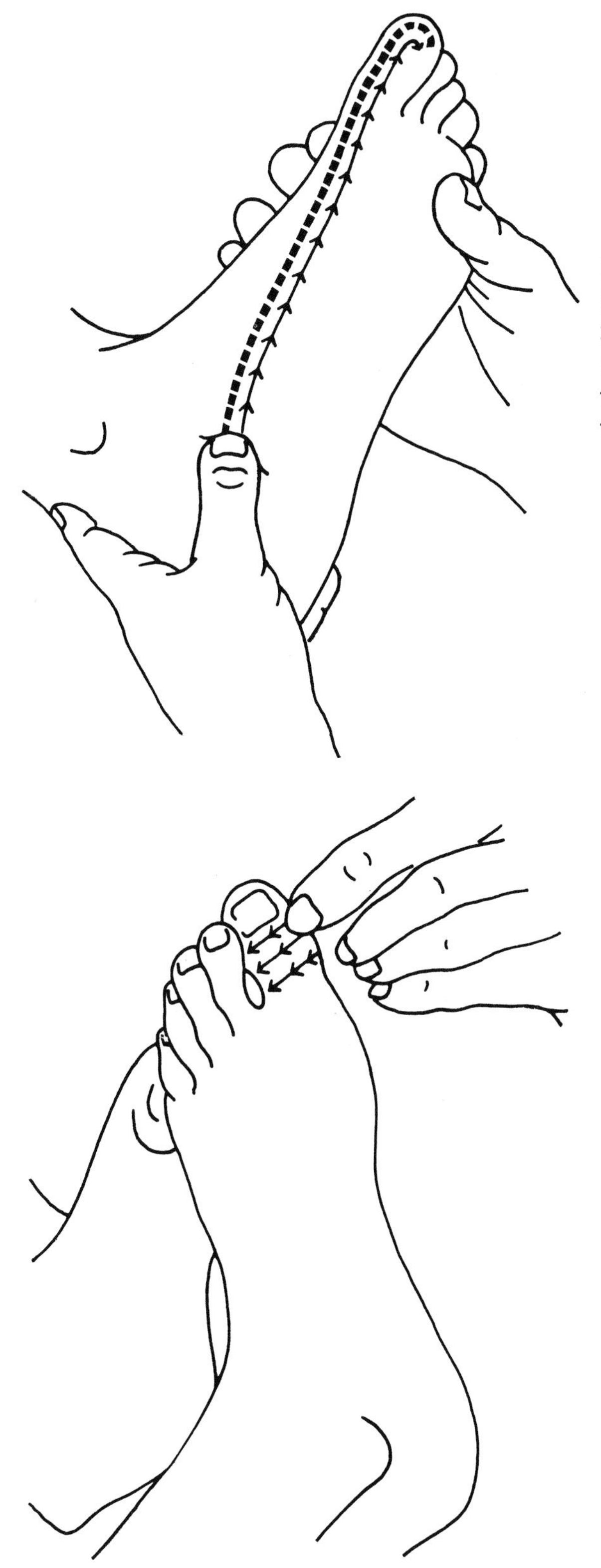

Figure 10.13 The spinal cord and brain (left foot), zones 1 2 3.
Supporting the left foot with the right hand and using the left thumb, work up the spine and into the brain area two or three times.

Figure 10.14 Facial area (left foot), zone 1.
Supporting the left foot with your right fist and using your left index finger, work across the big toe two or three times.

Case study: Brain damage

I am becoming increasingly interested in the usefulness of reflexology in treating brain-damaged children. I feel that if treatment could be conducted as soon after the disability is detected – and I really mean early – with frequent treatments from a trained practitioner as well as the parents being trained to stimulate the spine and brain area themselves (thus treating the child at least twice a day), there should be some very good results. In the whole of my career, I have only been able to work on two brain-damaged young children who came for a long period of time; in each case an excellent result was achieved. A young girl who stands vividly in my memory had minor brain damage at birth and although she was completely normal mentally, her right arm was totally paralysed and she dragged her right leg, which caused her to have many falls. Medically, all that could have been done for her had been done. She had had extensive physiotherapy, hydrotherapy, exercises, and very good supportive parents who encouraged as much movement and independence as could be achieved. She attended my surgery every week, and I asked her parents if she could remain with me for at least a year. I felt sure that by constantly stimulating the spine and the brain area there should be some spark of energy that could be encouraged, in order to improve the child's condition.

This little girl made a quite remarkable recovery; the disability was much reduced – in fact, walking became near normal, but unfortunately she did not gain the use in her right arm. Her parents did as I asked, treated her twice-daily, and with a weekly full treatment from me, including body massage, they were quite delighted with the result.

The pelvis is much stronger than the shoulder girdle as it has to support the full weight of the body. The spinal column is very much like cotton reels upon a rope, and the spine itself has tremendous abilities for movement. We can bend forwards, backwards, to the right, to the left and rotate our head upon our neck. The spine consists of seven cervical, twelve thoracic and five lumbar bones and the five sacral and four vertebrae of the coccyx together form a 'tail' which does not protrude from the body.

The thorax consists of twelve pairs of ribs articulating with the thoracic vertebrae, ten pairs joined with a cartilaginous process to the sternum in the front, leaving the two lowest pairs 'floating'. All bones have an outer, compact, sense layer and inner spongy cancellous centre. This makes them strong and light. They also act as storage for calcium and phosphorus. The articulating surfaces of the body are covered with cartilage to supply a smooth surface for the joint. There is no nerve supply to the bone, but blood vessels enter through the nutrient canal to reach the cancellous centre.

Growth takes place in all bones, but is more obviously apparent in long bones. All bones are formed from cartilage with the exception of the clavicle, and some of the skull, which ossify directly from the membrane.

The lumbar vertebrae are much denser and stronger than the thoracic vertebrae because the whole weight of the body is supported from this section.

The thoracic vertebrae are finer and have less density as they are not weight-bearing, and they only have to support the structure of the rib cage. The cervical vertebrae are finer and less dense as they only have to support the weight of the skull. The atlas and axis are two special vertebrae at the very top of the skull. The axis allows rotation of the head and the atlas allows nodding.

A joint is a meeting point of bones. It usually allows a controlled amount of movement. Some joints have to be very strong, while others tend to be very mobile. It is not possible for a joint to be strong and mobile, because they have to be able to withstand the friction of movement. The surfaces of bone are covered with smooth cartilage. The joint edge has a strong, fibrous capsule surrounding a sac of synovial membrane between the bone ends. This membrane secretes a small amount of lubricant fluid that allows frictionless movement, and the anti-articular cartilage keeps the two bones apart. The joint has stabilising ligaments which bind and strengthen it. There are different types of joint: a saddle joint allows movement in two directions but without rotation, for example ankle and thumb joints between wrist bones and thumb; hinge joints allow extension and flexion, for example elbow and finger joints; plane joints, where flat surfaces allow the bones to slide on each other, but they are restricted by ligaments to a small range, for example tarsal bones of the foot and between the ribs and thoracic vertebrae. There are also ball-and-socket joints: a joint freely moving in all directions, such as shoulder and hip joints. Pivot joints allow rotation but no other movement – as between the atlas and axis in the neck.

The spine – discs

The main joints between the vertebrae of the spine are slightly mobile. The vertebral surface is covered with hyaline cartilage and the intervening space is filled with a thick ring of fibrous cartilage with a centre of soft, almost gelatinous tissue. The joints are held together by the anterior and posterior longitudinal ligaments and muscles.

The spinal vertebrae also have joints between their other articulating surfaces on the neural arches and with the ribs in the thoracic region. These have a synovial membrane and are surrounded by ligaments. This allows a much greater degree of movement. The joints between the atlas and occiput and between the axis and atlas do not have discs but rely on synovial membranes to give movement. The intervertebral discs act as shock absorbers. The movement between the individual vertebrae, with the exception of the axis and atlas, is small, but the overall combining effect is considerable.

Most of the flexion and extension is in the cervical and lumbar regions; bending to the side is principally in the thoracic area. Twisting involves the whole vertebral column. The intervertebral discs tend to wear through the years, and can eventually become as thin as a crisp. This probably explains why old people become shorter because, if they lose spaces between the discs through wear and tear, they are obviously going to become shorter as they get older and dehydration occurs. The statement which is common on results from X-rays – 'narrowing of the disc space' – means just that.

How reflexology can help

There are obviously limitations in what we can achieve in degenerative conditions of the spine in the elderly, but generally reflexology can offer some reduction in pain and stiffness.

The reflex points to the spine are absolutely vital in the treatment of reflexology. As nerves arise out of the cranial and spinal regions, it is quite obvious that there are stimulations through nerve pathways to all organs and functions of the body through the spine. If you only have twenty minutes to help a friend who is generally feeling unwell and may be suffering from some aches and pains in the body, working for at least ten minutes up and down the spinal area via the feet will give her a tremendous uplift in her health and relief from pain. However, this short treatment is only to be used in extreme circumstances and in an instance where a complete treatment session is just not possible.

There are many back conditions that are common today, and the general medical treatment for back pain is normally pain-killing medications, anti-inflammatory drugs, and in many instances complete bed rest. Physiotherapy is often advised, and in many cases this does eventually solve the problem.

However, reflexology has proved to be of immense benefit to problems relating to the back. All sorts of conditions, from lumbago to sciatica, frozen shoulders, whiplash injuries which affect both the neck and the lumbar spinal area, have all responded admirably to reflexology treatment. In fact, I would say that reflexologists treat more patients with back conditions than any other form of health problem. I am also happy to say that the benefits we achieve in treating back conditions are very great. Reflexology has the benefit of breaking down inflammatory states giving relief and freedom to the ligaments and muscles, which undoubtedly go into spasm, and improving the nerve and blood supply to the spine.

The vertebral column of the spine and the central nervous system share exactly the same reflex points within the foot, as the spinal cord actually extends from the foramen magnum, a hole in the base of the skull, to the second lumbar vertebrae.

Back conditions are on the increase and this is due mainly to the fact that man has grown so much in a very short period of time. It was not very long ago when a man of average height could walk quite freely through the door of a small country cottage. It's hardly possible for anybody to be able to walk through these low doorways now. Our teenagers are growing to be quite tall due in the main to the decrease in infant disease. Rickets and rheumatic fever are, thankfully, a thing of the past and the great improvement in nutrition and the care and welfare of infants is quite considerable, particularly in this country. Generally speaking, the taller you are the more likely you will be to suffer from back conditions, simply because the spine has more to support. A person with a shorter, more squat body structure has less trouble with their spine. Also, another of the big causes of back conditions is the fact that people do not exercise nearly enough. The muscle tone of the abdomen and the spine itself are vital in the support of the spinal structure. Sitting in cars for long periods of time is not an advantage to the spine, particularly when both our feet are poised in an unusual position and the weight of our spine is centred onto the lumbar region. What normally happens is that we tend to sit about in cars, in our homes and in offices during the week and then spend the weekends exerting ourselves excessively. For instance, we play a fast game of squash or dig in the garden, only to find that the following day we are hardly able to move.

Many pains in the knees are as the result of a lumbar spinal problem. It is often quite amazing how extreme pain in the knee, either due to an arthritic condition or something even worse, reveals in an X-ray no damage whatsoever, and the sensitivity being experienced which is completely disabling has been caused through compression through the lumbar spinal vertebrae. One of the great benefits of reflexology is the ability to be able to find out within the foot whence the source of trouble came. The causative area is the one that reveals sensitivity to the patient; that is, the patient will react and exclaim that the area upon which you are at present working is extremely sensitive – and this is the source of the cause of the condition that you are treating.

The feet never lie. When there is a sensitivity in the foot it always denotes a problem in the physical body.

We are also able to treat frozen shoulders most successfully, and reflexology helps admirably with freeing tension and pain in cases of arthritis.

Tennis elbow is another condition which frequently comes to our surgeries and reflexology is able to give a lot of relief here as well. Chronic neck inflammations, as in cases of arthritis of the cervical spine, or the damage caused by a whiplash injury, are common conditions and can be eased with reflexology treatment.

One of the most agonising conditions associated with the spine is sciatica. It can become so acute that the patient is hardly able to use their leg. Although it does take quite a long period of treatments we do have good results in coping with sciatica.

Practical procedures for working the skeletal system

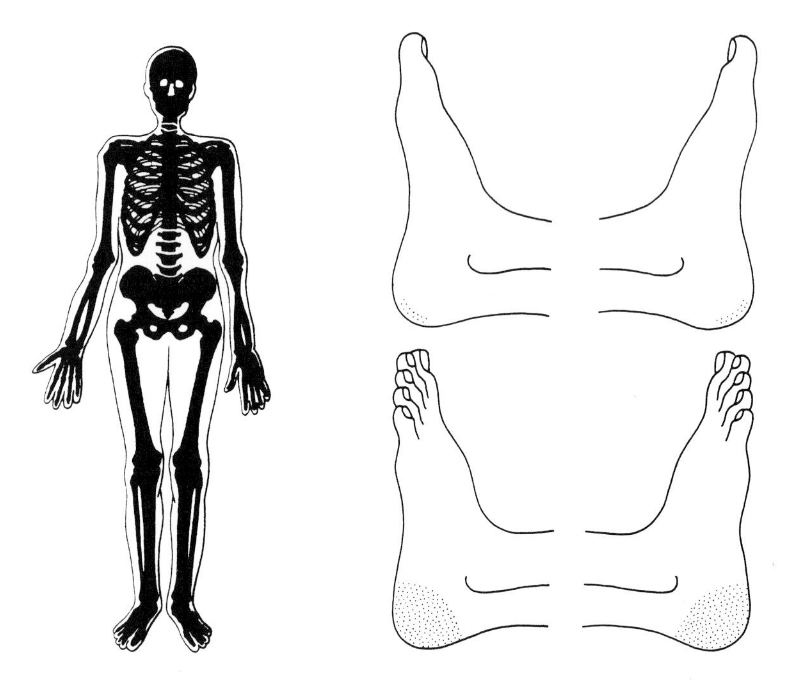

Figure 11.2 Areas relating to (a) the coccyx, hip and pelvis

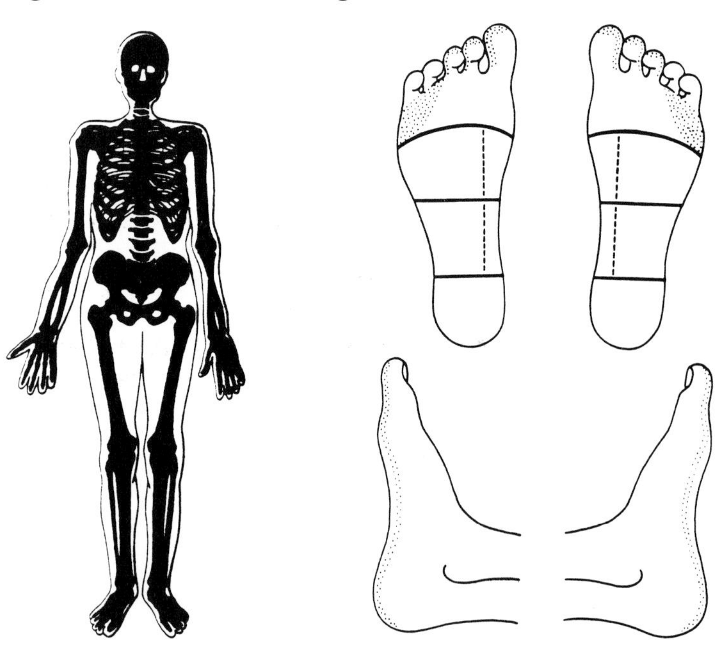

(b) the spine, neck, brain and shoulder

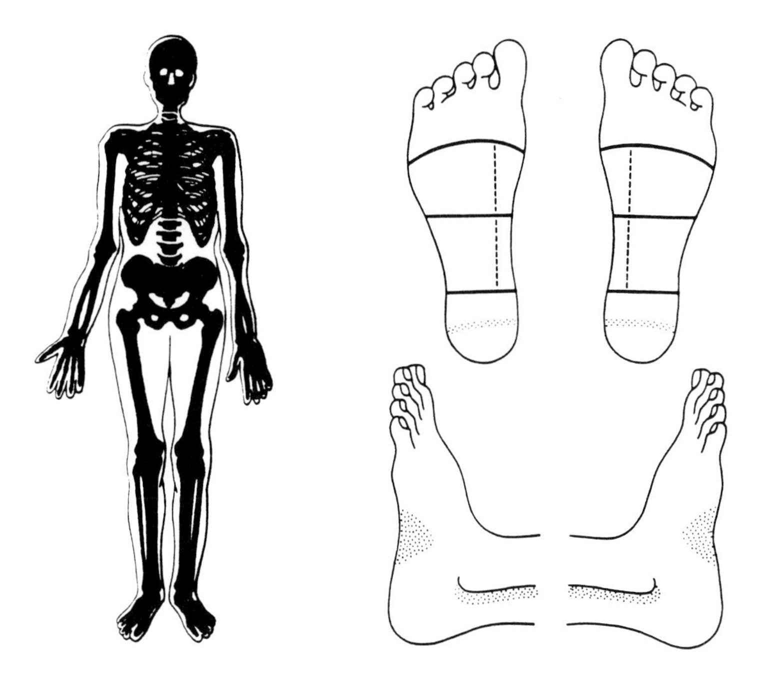

(c) the primary and secondary sciatic area, knee and elbow

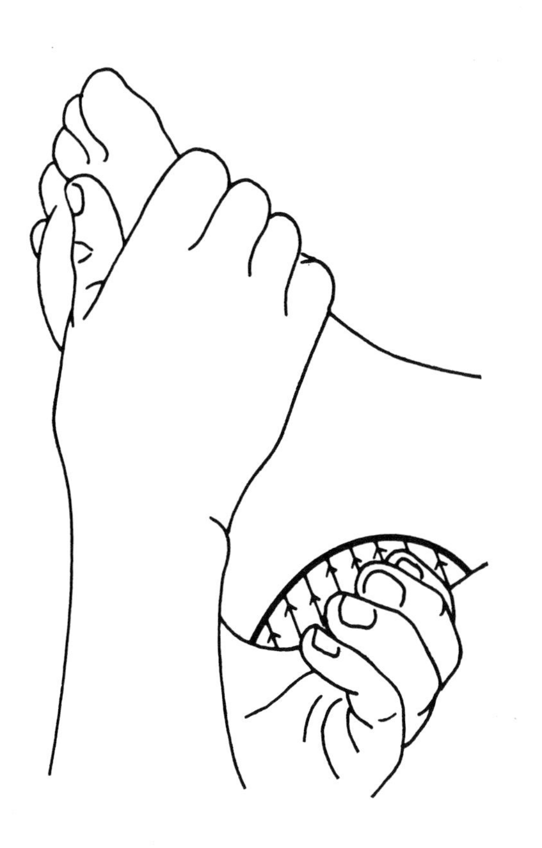

Figure 11.3 The vertebral column (right foot), working out the area to the coccyx, zone 1, support medial.
Holding the medial side of the right foot with your right hand, use pressure from the four fingers of your left hand. Repeat this procedure two or three times.

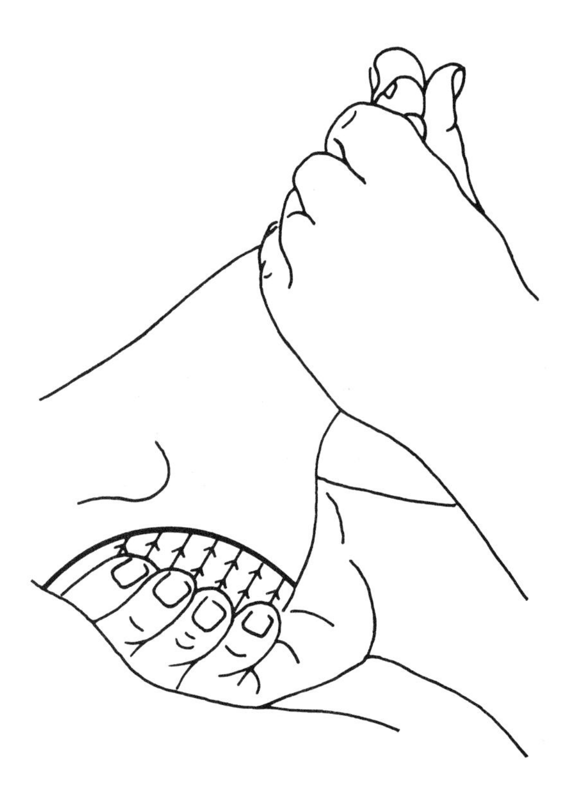

Figure 11.4 The vertebral column (right foot), working out the area to the hip/ pelvis, zone 5, support lateral. Supporting the right foot with your left hand, use pressure from the four fingers of your right hand. Repeat this procedure two or three times.

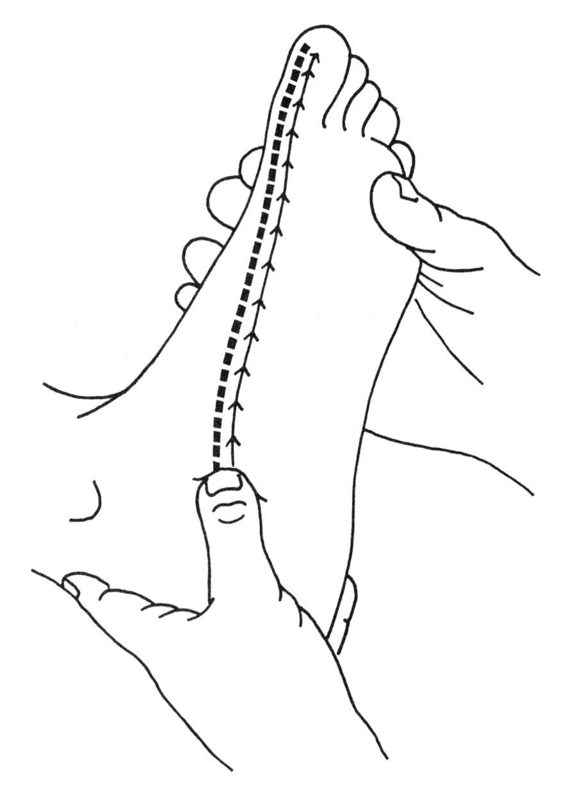

Figure 11.5 The vertebral column (left foot), working out the area of the vertebral column, zone 1, support top. Supporting the left foot with your right hand and using the left thumb, proceed to work up the vertebral column.

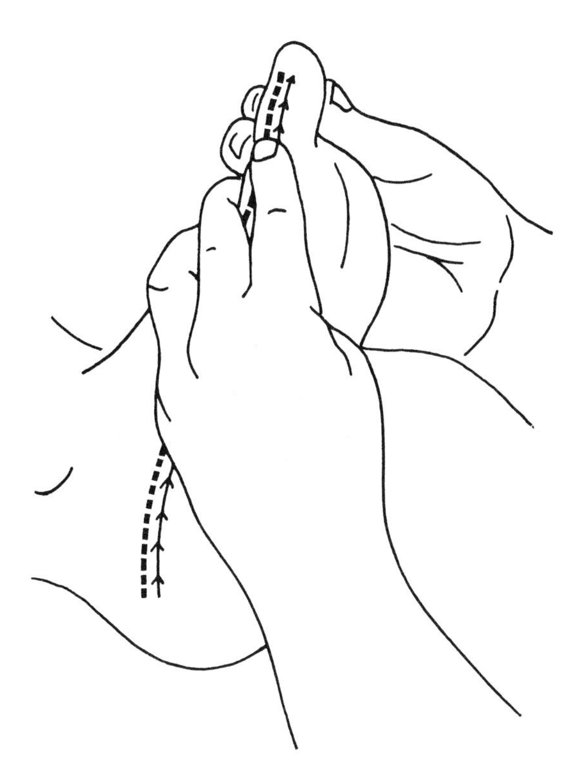

Figure 11.6 The vertebral column (left foot), working out the area of the cervical spine, zone 1, support top.
Supporting the left foot with your right hand and using the left index finger, proceed to work up the very fine area of the cervical spine. (A better result will be achieved with the index finger.)

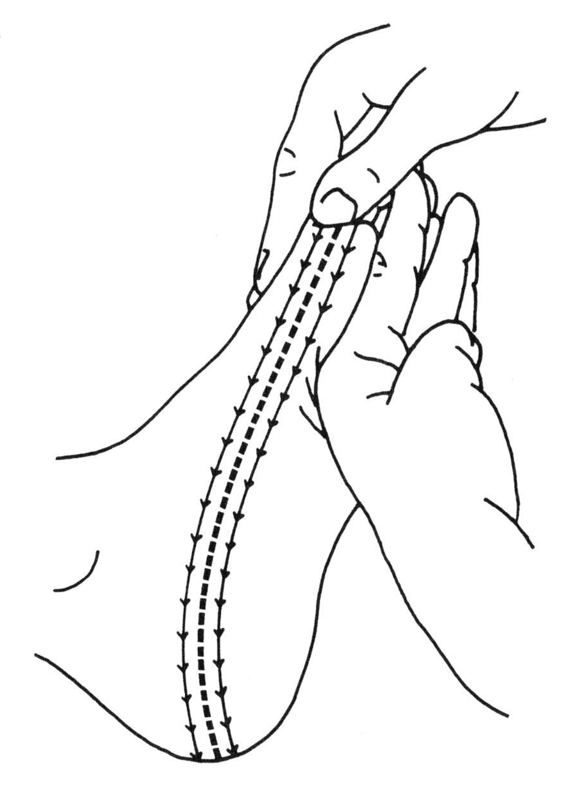

Figure 11.7 The vertebral column (left foot), working down the vertebral column.
Supporting the left foot with the flat of your left hand, work down the vertebral column with the thumb of your right hand.

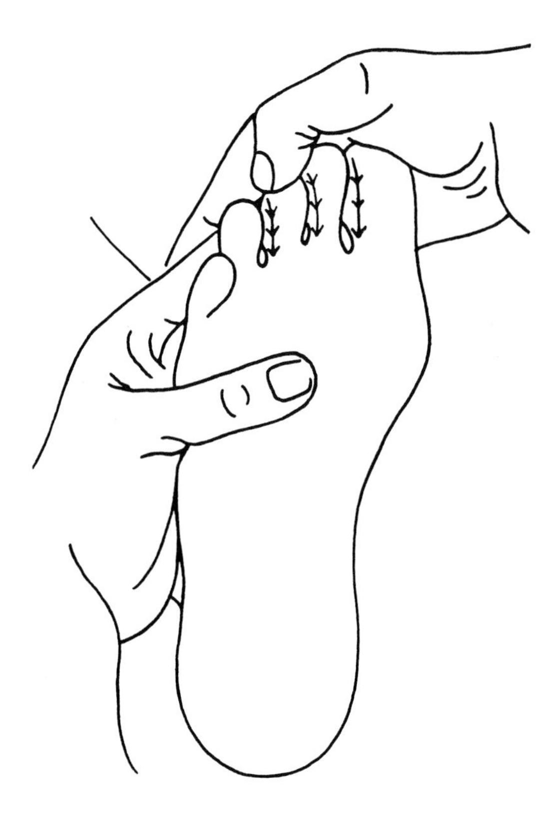

Figure 11.8 The chronic neck (right foot), working out the areas of the chronic neck, zones 1 2 3, support top.
Supporting the right foot with your left hand, proceed to work down the lateral sides of the first three toes with your right thumb.

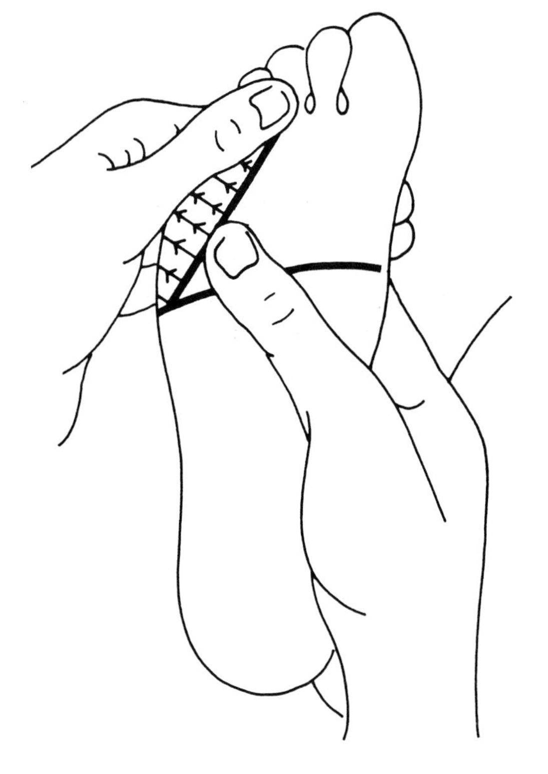

Figure 11.9 Shoulder area (right foot), plantar view, zones 4 and 5, medial to lateral.
Supporting the right foot with your left hand, work out the area from medial to lateral with your right thumb.

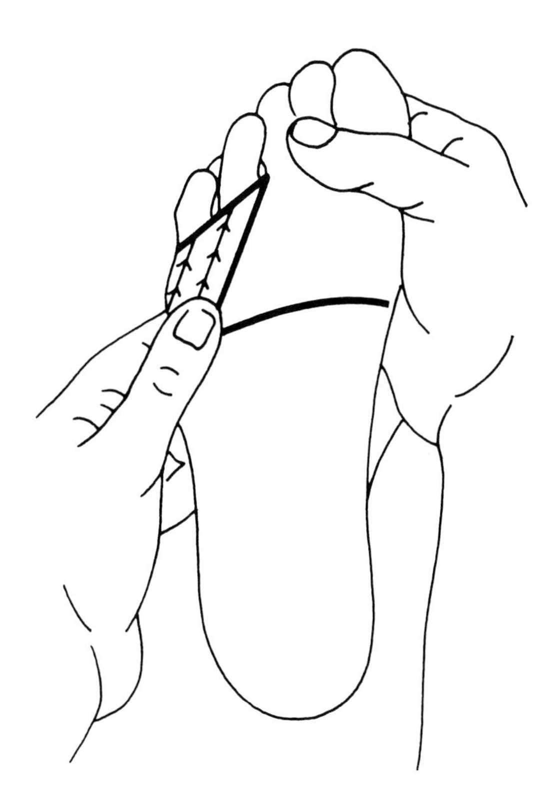

Figure 11.10 Shoulder area (right foot), plantar view, zones 4 and 5, lateral to medial.
Supporting the right foot with your right hand, work out the area from lateral to medial with your left thumb.

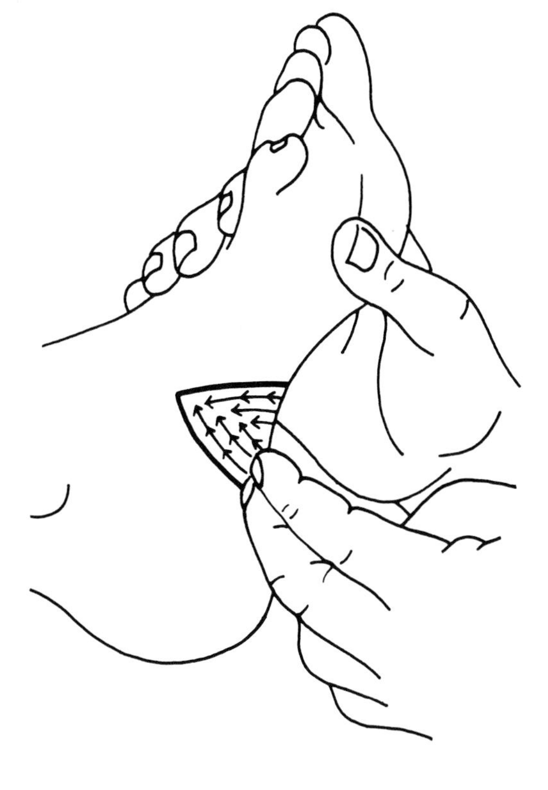

Figure 11.11 Knee/elbow area (right foot), zone 5, top support.
Supporting the right foot with your right hand and using your left index finger, work out the entire triangular area.

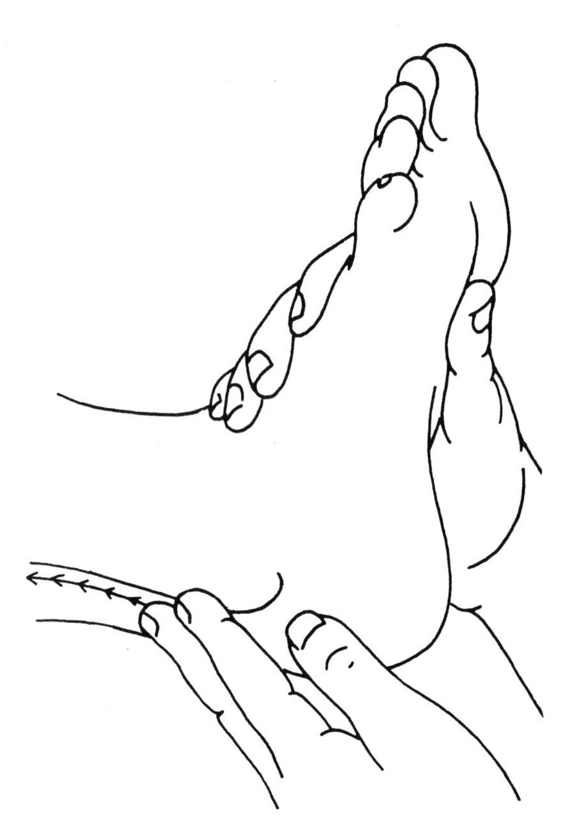

Figure 11.12 Primary sciatic area (right foot), lateral view, zone 5, top support. Supporting the right foot with your right hand and using pressure from the index and third finger of your left hand, work up the area just behind the ankle bone. Proceed for about three inches.

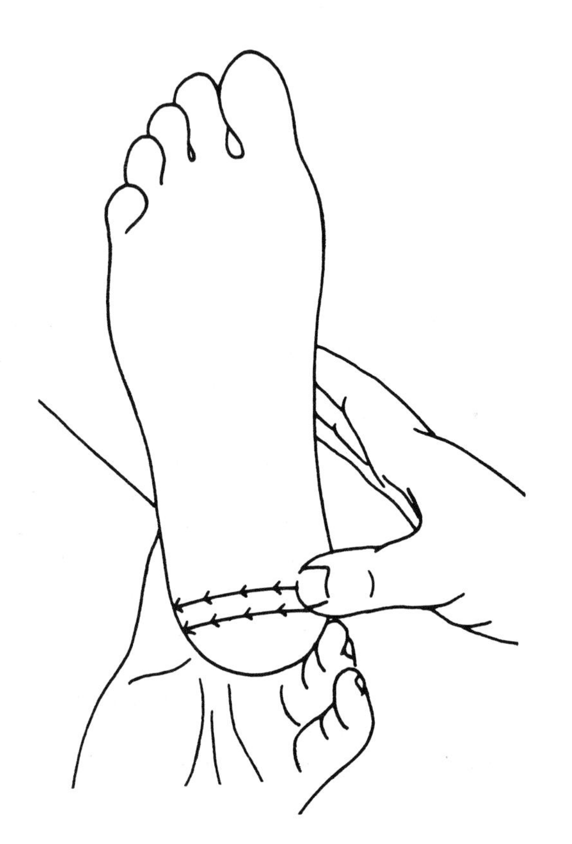

Figure 11.13 The secondary sciatic area (right foot), zones 1 2 3 4 5, medial to lateral, heel support.
Supporting the right foot in the palm of your left hand and using the right thumb, work out the area two or three times.

CHAPTER 12 The urinary system

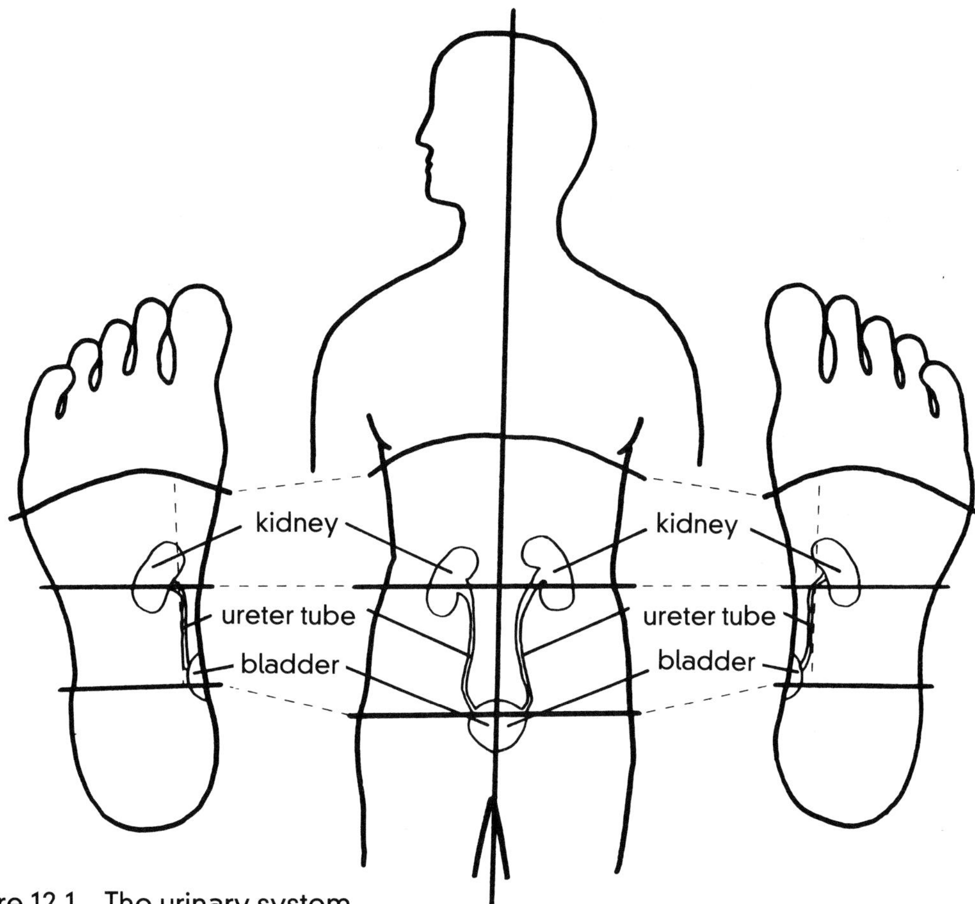

Figure 12.1 The urinary system

The urinary system comprises two kidneys, two ureter tubes and a bladder controlled by a sphincter muscle. The kidneys are a pair of organs for filtering impurities from the blood. They prevent poisons fatally accumulating in the body. The kidneys are two bean-shaped objects behind the stomach, one on each side of the spine, and together the kidneys are the same size as the heart.

The cortex and medulla contain tiny blood filtration units called nephrons. A single kidney has more than a million nephrons. Urine, the waste product of filtration, collects in the kidneys' pelvis. Blood for processing enters the medulla from the renal artery. Inside the medulla and cortex, the artery splits into tiny, coiled blood vessels. Each coiled blood vessel is called a glomerulus. Almost completely surrounding this lies a sac the size of a pin head called the Bowmans' capsule. Pressure forces water and dissolved chemicals from the blood in the glomerulus into the Bowmans' capsule. The filtered liquid then continues through a tubule surrounded by capillaries.

These tiny blood vessels reabsorb into the blood most of the water and useful chemicals such as amino acids. The treated blood then leaves the kidney via the renal vein.

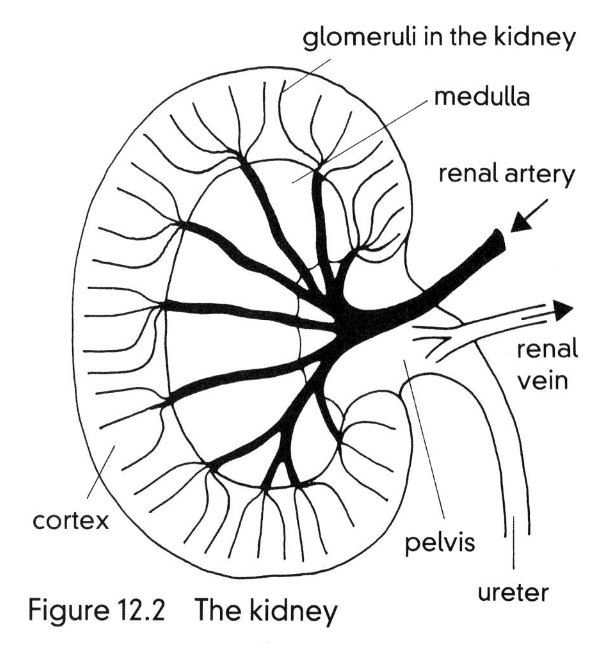

Figure 12.2 The kidney

Meanwhile, wastes remaining in the convoluted tubule flow on via a collecting tube to the kidneys' pelvis. These wastes now form urine, an amber liquid largely made of water, uric acid, urea and inorganic salts. From the kidneys' pelvis urine leaves the kidney through a tube known as the ureter. The urinary bladder stores urine before it leaves the body. It is a hollow, muscular bag lying just behind the hip bone called the pubis.

One pair of kidneys can process 190 litres (42 gallons) of blood a day. Urine output drops in sleep or during perspiration and rises after more liquid than usual has been drunk.

The two ureters connect the bladder to the kidneys. A broader tube, the urethra, opens from the bottom of the bladder. A ring of muscles called the urethral sphincter normally keeps this outlet closed.

An empty bladder is flat, a full bladder can hold about a pint of urine. Urine drips into the bladder through the ureter tubes and the bladder walls relax as it fills. When the bladder holds about a cup-full of urine, nerves start sending signals to the brain to urinate. Urination occurs when the urethral sphincter relaxes and the bladder wall contracts, forcing urine out through the urethra.

How reflexology can help

The types of conditions reflexologists are able to relieve include stress incontinence. A patient may find that, during episodes of physical stress – such as coughing, laughing or lifting heavy objects – urine is released against that person's will from the bladder. This condition can occur in women who have had several pregnancies or in the very elderly, whose bladder muscle function has become weakened with the ageing process. Good results have also been achieved with kidney stones. In some strange way, reflexology seems to enable the ureter tube to become more relaxed and to allow the stone to pass through into the bladder with the least discomfort. Reflexology can also be most effective in treating kidney conditions. Nephritis has been greatly relieved with frequent sessions, and cystitis, a common illness affecting far more women than men because the female urethra tube is much shorter than the males, has also been relieved.

Another illness closely associated with the kidneys is high blood pressure. Patients suffering from chronic hypertension often find that the kidney function can eventually become impaired. The increased pressure being forced through the kidney tubules often causes a collapse and less efficient function of the filtering system, so it is common to find that patients suffering from hypertension will have very sensitive reactions when the kidney reflexes are worked upon. By taking the stress off the kidney area, we are able in turn to improve the complete kidney function, and this has an effect on lowering the blood pressure.

It is very beneficial to work the areas connected to the pelvic hip and coccyx area and also the lumbar spine when treating bladder and kidney problems. I feel that by stimulating the whole pelvic cavity we are able to break down a lot of stress and tension, and help rid the body of impurities.

Practical procedures for working the urinary system

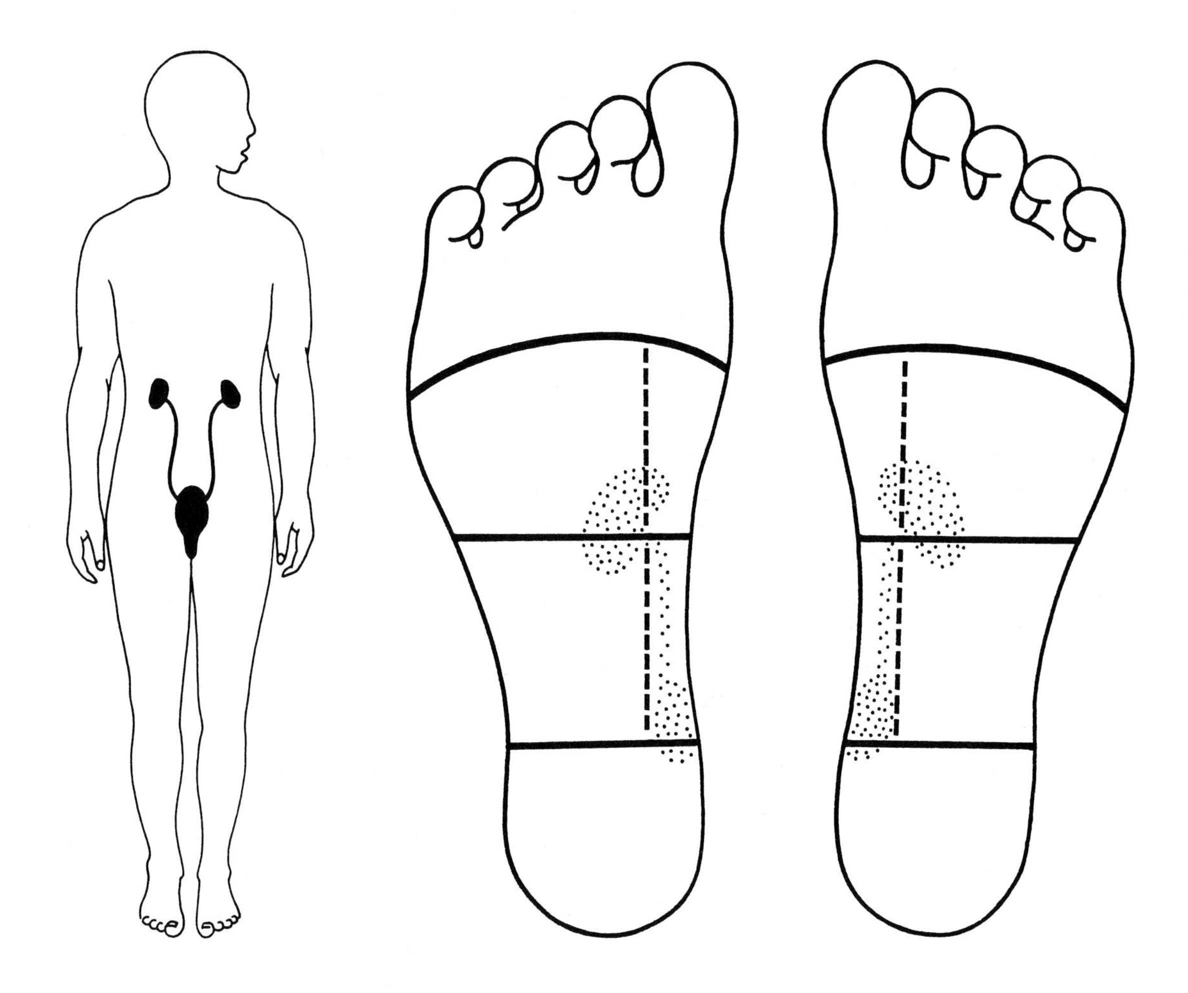

Figure 12.3 Areas relating to the urinary system

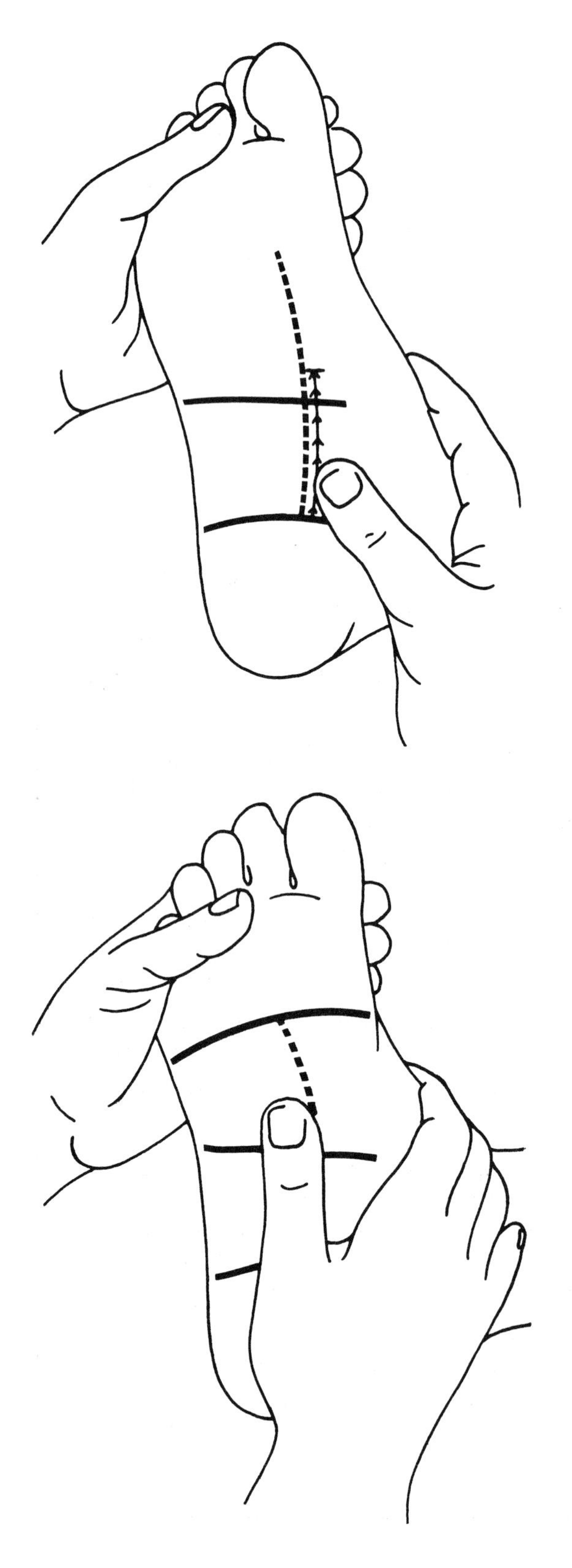

Figure 12.4 The bladder and ureter tube (right foot), zone 1, top support, medial. Supporting the right foot at the top with your left hand, work on and over the bladder area with the right thumb. Proceed up the medial side of the ligament line to work out the ureter tube.

Figure 12.5 The kidney (right foot), zone 2, top support, medial. Supporting the right foot with your left hand and placing the right thumb on the lateral side of the ligament line, work out the area as indicated.

Case study: Kidney pain

A particular case comes to mind as I write about the urinary system. This was a rather strange case where the feet, in a different way, expressed the irritation of problems within the body.

A woman came to me suffering from a very sore, irritated patch on the sole of her foot and this was positioned in the kidney reflex area. This sore patch was very like eczema; it was weepy and scaly, and the skin was red and sore.

This woman had been to a dermatologist and had had extensive X-rays to see if there was a foreign body lurking in the foot, but nothing had proved of any significance. She said that the main problem was that most of her nights were spent awake with this extremely irritating patch. No sooner had she got into bed and got warm than the patch became more inflamed, and she was constantly in and out of bed putting her foot in cold water and desperately trying to get some relief. All the creams and lotions she had applied only gave her a short relief and in desperation she decided to try a course of reflexology treatments.

I found it very difficult to understand why the eczema was in such a confined space on just one foot when in fact she had had no previous history of eczema. The symptoms were puzzling until I found, after taking an extensive case history, that in the past the patient had suffered from kidney stones which had caused a lot of damage to the right kidney. This area of the foot in fact was on the right, in the same area as the reflex to the kidney would be found. I felt that maybe this could be one of those exceptional cases where the irritation in the foot was expressing the damage to and inflammation of an organ, so it was therefore a reaction of a very different sort.

The main problem was how were we going to treat this area of the foot when the skin was so angry and inflamed; any contact with this point would have caused a lot of distress to the patient. I covered the area with a large piece of lint attached by some plaster and applied a very light pressure to this angry area. I also extensively worked out the bladder, ureter tube and kidney on the left foot, as I felt that maybe just general elimination would be helpful. I was restricted in the amount of time I could spend because of the discomfort in the area, but told the patient that I felt sure that we were on the right track and that if she could come back for a few sessions we would just see whether in fact the area started to heal. We could then work more extensively on the kidney reflex point on the right foot. On the second visit she said that she did feel that the irritation in that area had reduced and the skin didn't seem to be quite so inflamed, and so I was able to give her a more extensive treatment. She reported that after her second treatment she experienced sharp pains in her right kidney area – the right kidney area in the body, not in the foot. I then knew that we were on the right track.

A further six sessions of treatment resulted in the healing of the inflamed, damaged area of the foot. After most treatment sessions, and occasionally during them as well, she also confirmed to me that she now realised that she often experienced a sharp reaction of pain in her kidney area on the right side. At the end of the treatment all inflammation in the foot was completely healed, the frequency of pain in the kidney area didn't return and the patient made a full recovery.

Case study: Kidney stones

A further interesting case that comes to mind was that of a middle-aged man who came to me with a history of kidney stones. This problem had troubled him for many years, and every few months he had excruciating pain in the low back area. He experienced a lot of bleeding and laceration of the tubules in the kidney, which caused retention of urine and, eventually, after these episodes had subsided he would pass one or two kidney stones. The pain during these episodes was so intense that he had to call his doctor out to visit him, and he was usually given an injection of morphine. There was no real help that medicine could offer and he just limped along with his routine and came to me eventually through an introduction from a friend.

His treatment session revealed great sensitivity in both the left kidney area and, extensively, in the ureter tube and the left kidney. I certainly felt that the diagnosis of damage and scarring to the kidney was very obvious. I proceeded to treat this patient weekly. The morning after the first session, he rang to say that, much to his amazement, in the evening after the treatment (which was in the early afternoon), he had sharp pains in his left kidney area, and later in the evening passed several small kidney stones with associated bleeding, but the most surprising thing of all was that he did not suffer the agonising pain of the past. I felt that in some uncanny way reflexology had eased the tension in the kidney and ureter area and enabled the kidney stones to be passed through with less tension.

This patient continued treatment, and exactly the same reaction occurred after every treatment. In a few hours he would pass one or two kidney stones, but without the associated discomfort. After six treatments his condition seemed to have improved and he stopped passing kidney stones. He said he'd lost all pain and sensation in this area, and agreed that he would stop treatment for the next few months and just see how he proceeded. He was very well for a further nine months and then reported similar symptoms again, and so back he came for some further treatments when exactly the same procedures occurred.

Reflexology was not able to cease the production of kidney stones in this man, but what it was able to do was to lessen the discomfort and give him great relief. In the long term it was able to reduce the episodes of pain and discomfort. This patient still returns occasionally with similar symptoms, but the gaps are getting longer and I feel sure that his improvement is totally due to the benefits of reflexology.

CHAPTER 13 The reproductive system

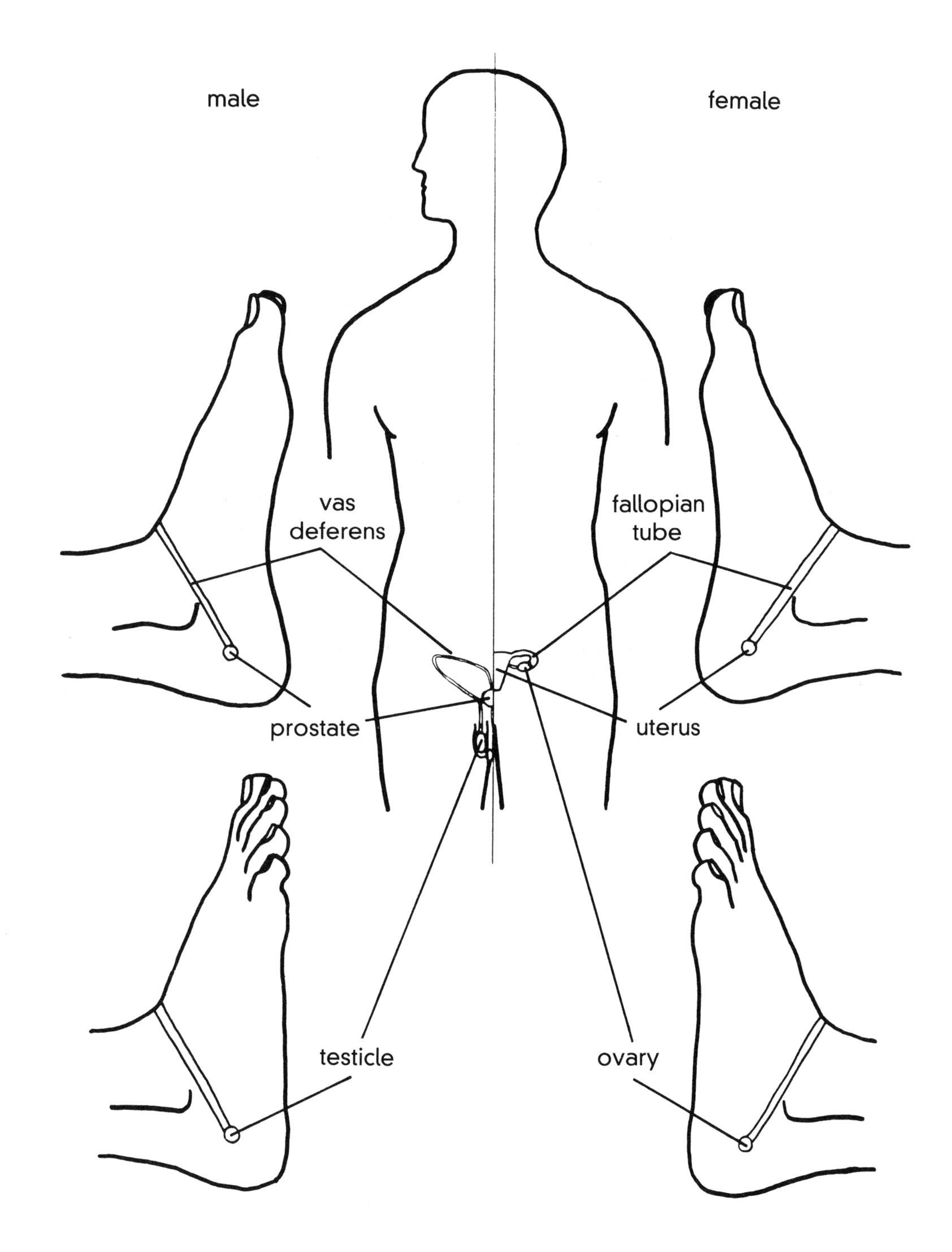

Figure 13.1 The reproductive system

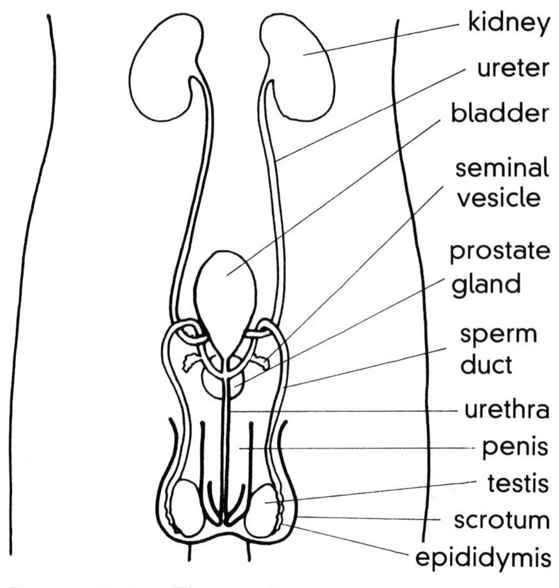

Figure 13.2 The male reproductive organs

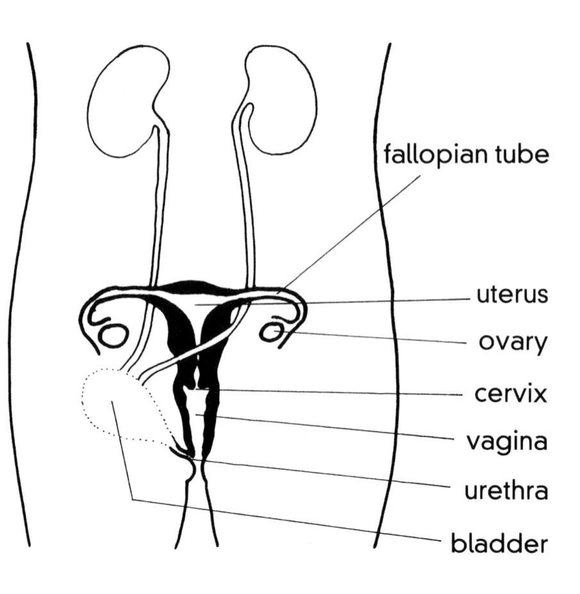

Figure 13.3 The female reproductive organs

Male anatomy

The reproductive system comprises in the male two testes, which hang in the scrotal sac, the vasa efferentia which joins the testis to the overlying epididymis, and the vas deferens, which joins the urethra in the centre of the prostate gland. The seminal vesicle acts as a storage organ for the mature sperm.

The prostate gland lies around the first part of the urethra at the base of the bladder, and its secretions help maintain sperm activity. Two additional pairs of glands, Cowper's and Littre's, empty into the urethra adjacent to the prostate. They produce the bulk of the ejaculate of three to five millilitres of semen.

The penis is the male organ of reproduction. It also has another function, which is the excretion of urine from the bladder out of the body.

The testes

Testes have two functions: the production of testosterone and of spermatoza. The tubules produce large quantities of sperm every day which pass into a series of communicating ducts. These ducts, lined with cells, join to form twelve to twenty vasa efferentia which run to the epididymis where the sperm spends up to ten days maturing before entering the vas deferens. Testosterone responds to the luteinizing hormone. It causes development of male secondary sexual characteristics – pubic and facial hair growth, aggressiveness, muscle bulk and deepening of the voice.

Female anatomy

The female reproductive system not only has to produce an ovum but it also has to provide nutrition to the fertilised ovum and protect it until pregnancy ends. At the entrance to the vagina are a pair of lip-like folds – the larger and thicker being the labia majora, and the smaller, inner fold being the labia minora. They lie along either side of the vaginal entrance and join in the front, blending into the padded area of the mons pubis. At the front, they enclose the exit of the urethra just behind the small projection of tissue, the clitoris, which is comparable to the penis.

Behind these structures is the vagina, a 10–15cm elastic tube lined with moist epithelium. At the top of the vagina the uterus is held in place by muscles and four strong, fibrous ligaments of the pelvic floor, and to the side of the pelvis by pairs of round and suspensory ligaments running in folds of peritoneum.

The uterus is a small, pear-shaped organ covered with peritoneum with a thick wall of interweaving muscle fibres and lined with special endometrial cells. It is situated behind the bladder in front of the rectum. The cervix of the uterus is a thick, fibrous, muscular structure opening into the vagina and lined with special cells that form a 'plug' of mucus. Uterine muscles are always contracting and relaxing slightly. The two fallopian tubes are about 10cm long with finger-like fimbriae at the end to encircle the ovaries. The ovum is swept down the tube by a combination of ciliated epithelium and peristaltic muscular contraction.

Unlike the male urinary system, that of the female is separate from the reproductive system. The bladder empties into the urethra, which opens in front of the vagina.

The ovaries

The ovaries have two functions, the production of ova and secretion of oestrogen and progesterone. At puberty, the onset of menstruation and the development of the secondary sexual characteristics – hair growth, breast development and redistribution of fat to the buttocks and shoulders – are the result of the effect on the ovaries of the increasing pituitary secretion of follicle stimulation hormones (FSH) and luteinizing hormones (LH). The ovary contains 50 to 250,000 ovum, but only about 500 eventually become mature ova.

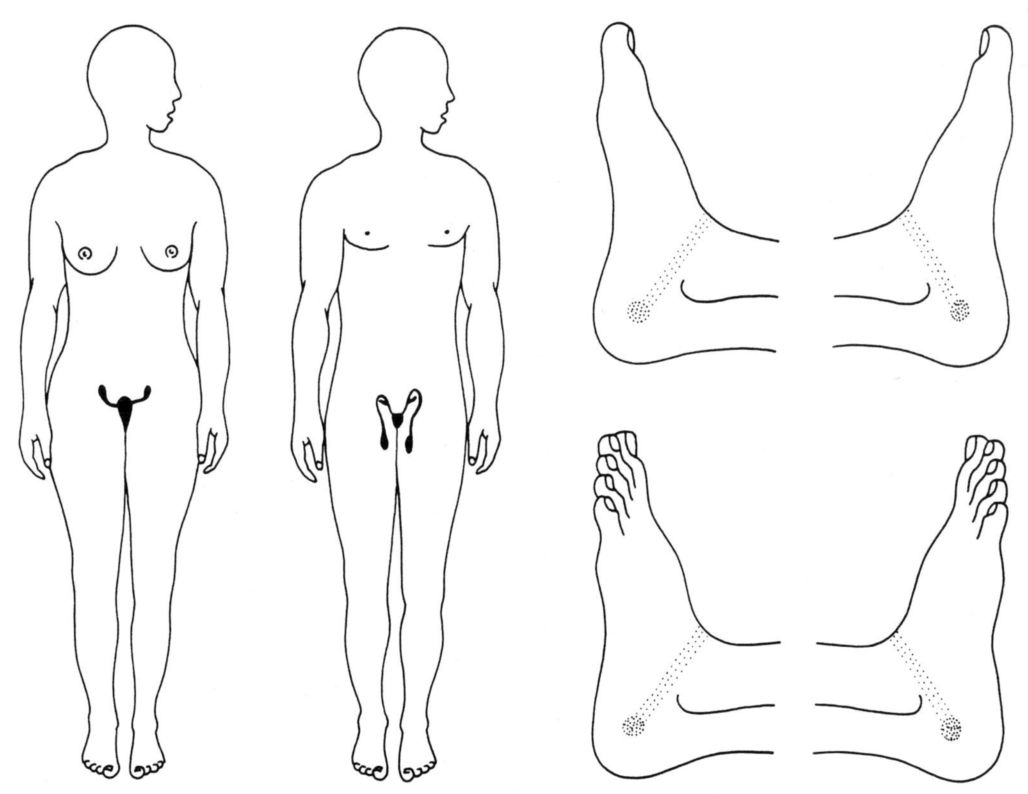

Figure 13.4 Areas relating to the male and female reproductive areas

Practical procedures for working the reproductive system

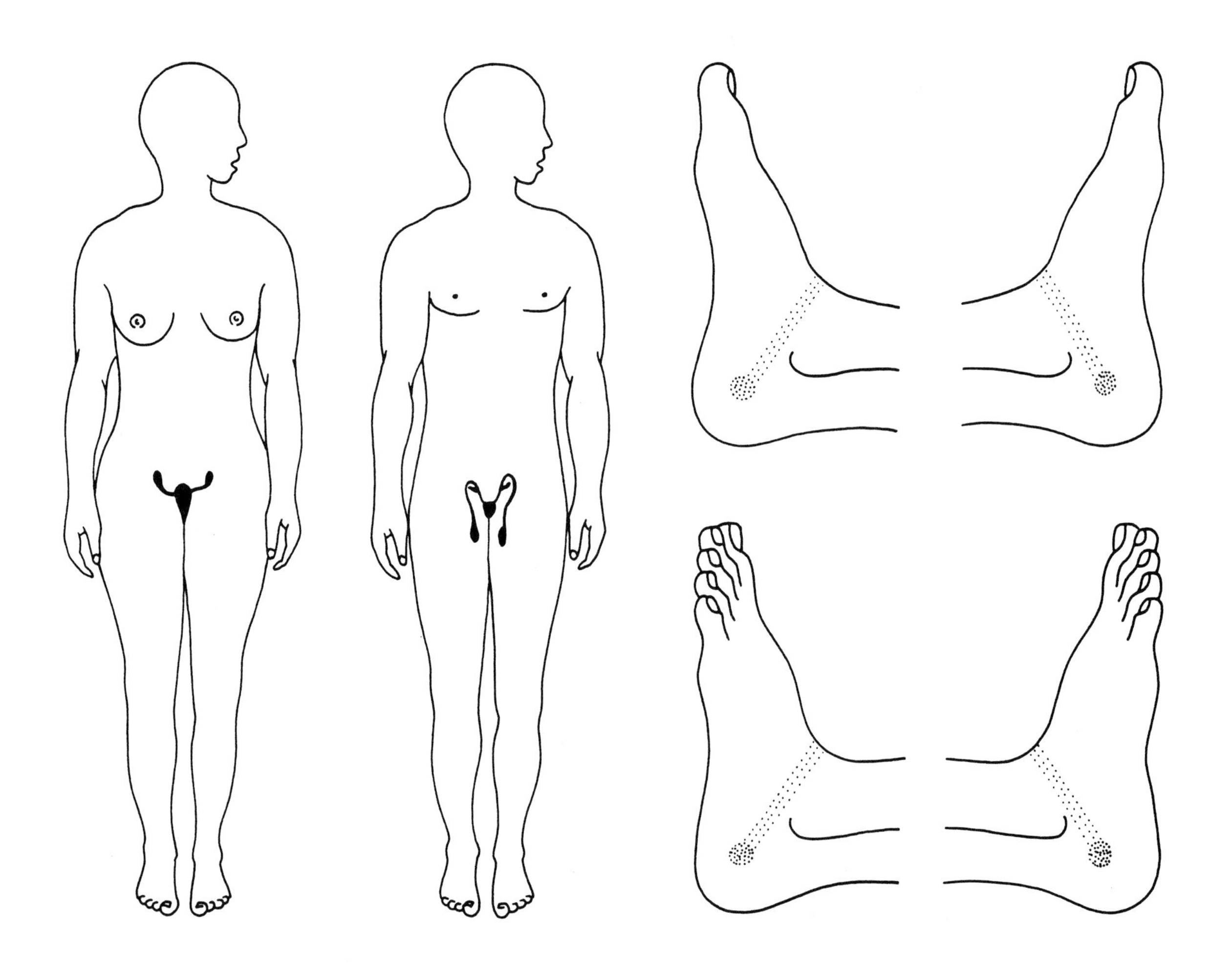

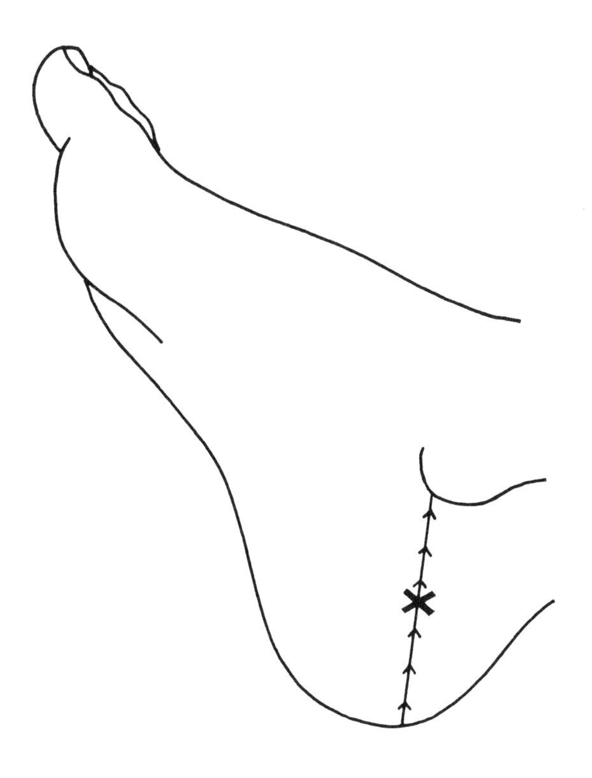

Figure 13.5 The uterus/prostate area (right foot), zone 1, medial.
These areas are to be found halfway between the ankle bone and the tip of the heel.

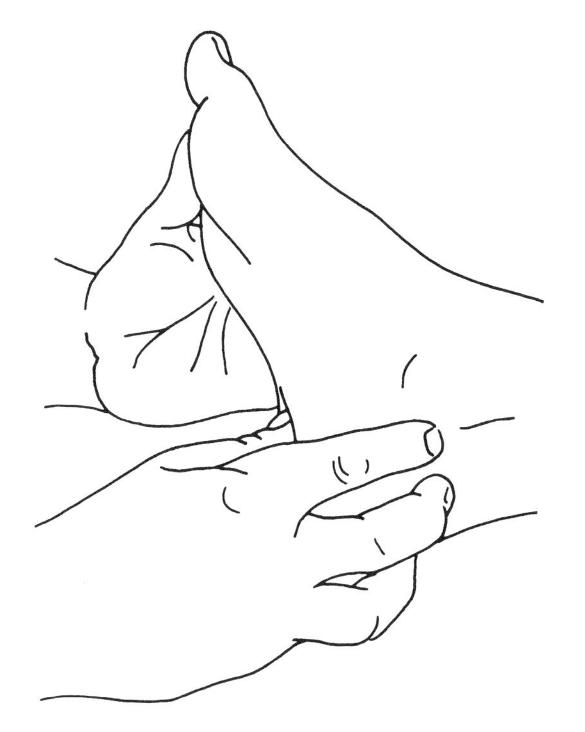

Figure 13.6 The uterus/prostate area (right foot).
Supporting the right foot with your left hand and using the right index finger, work in a straight line as identified in Figure 13.5. Repeat two or three times.

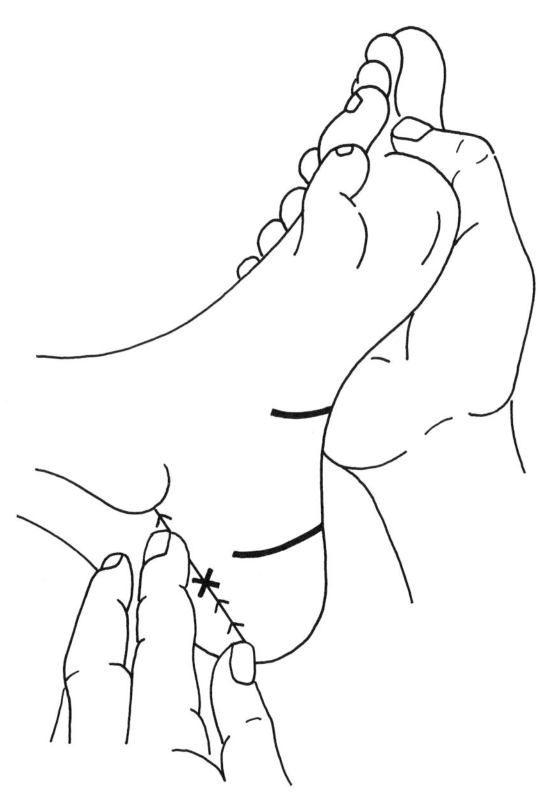

Figure 13.7 The ovary/testes (right foot), zone 5, heel support, lateral.
Supporting the right foot with your right hand and using the left index finger, work in a straight line two or three times.

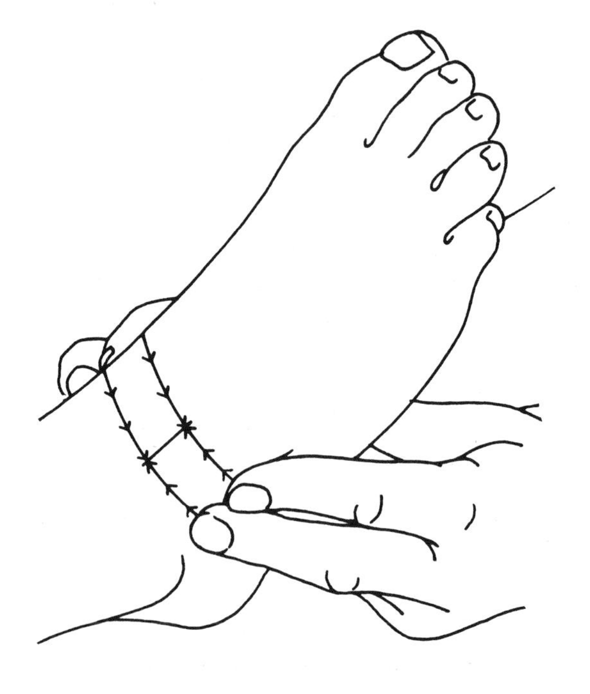

Figure 13.8 Fallopian tube/vas deferens (right foot).
Supporting from the plantar side of the foot, and pressing in for support with both thumbs, work around the front of the foot with the index and third finger together. Repeat two or three times.

CHAPTER 14 Drug reactions and areas of assistance

Drug reactions

It is essential to have an understanding of the side effects of a variety of drugs that are used in controlling symptoms and pain in various conditions.

Shortly after I started my practice, some eighteen years ago, I often used to pick up a sensitivity in the foot which did not really seem to relate to the condition that I was treating. As an example, I would be treating a patient for severe hay fever and would pick up extreme sensitivity in the sinus and lung-related areas of the foot which I expected, but I would then find that the kidney area was extremely sensitive. This was confusing: what on earth had the kidneys to do with hay fever? As the months went by there would be more and more queries. Sensitivities appeared in the feet which just did not link up to the problem the patient had come to me with. Maybe the chart which I was using was incorrect. Or was there something about reflexology which I had not been taught? Perhaps I would have to try and work this out for myself.

I noted that patients presenting with these various odd sensitivities were all on medications of some kind or another, and eventually, after consulting an encyclopaedia of drugs, I realised that what in fact I was picking up were congested areas in the body caused by the medications that the patient was taking.

As we all know, drugs have side effects, and cause inflammation and congestion and upset the functioning of other parts of the body. I list below some everyday drugs and the effect they have on the body.

Drugs – their side effects on the feet

The following drugs can create sensitivities in the reflexes to the organs on the feet.

Aspirin Commonly used to kill pain; creates stomach inflammation and sometimes stomach ulceration.

Anti-histamine Commonly used for allergic reactive illnesses, i.e. skin rashes, hay fever, troublesome irritant coughs and eczema. Anti-histamines create an inflammation in the kidney reflex area of the foot.

Antibiotics Commonly used to control infections in the body. They destroy the flora content in the intestine which upsets the balance of the body and can either cause constipation or diarrhoea. The liver is always affected when these drugs are used.

Anti-depressant drugs/sleeping pills These types of medication cause great sensitivity in the brain area of the foot.

Steroids Frequently used to break down inflammation and therefore commonly used for arthritis, heart conditions, cancer, severe allergic reactive illness such as asthma, which is uncontrollable. Taking steroids can create an insensitivity in the foot; therefore, you are likely to find no reaction at all, but it is worth while giving treatment as it still has an effect upon the body. Steroids lower a person's vitality.

Amphetamines These drugs are used in an attempt to reduce appetite for weight control. They are extremely addictive and stimulate all functioning of the body to work overtime, thereby creating a drastic effect on the central nervous system. The brain and adrenal glands are usually very sensitive in people taking this drug.

Beta-blockers Used in the control of heart conditions and hypertension. They dull down the sensitivity of the body and thus work as a depressant to the adrenal gland and heart. Therefore, the heart beat becomes lower. They have an effect on the liver.

Antacids Medications for digestive disturbances such as Rennies or any of those peppermint chalk-based medications. The chalk content in this medication has an effect upon the kidney, and if taken in large quantities over a long period of time, can cause kidney stones.

Painkillers All painkilling drugs do have a disastrous effect on the intestine, and normally cause chronic constipation.

Anti-inflammatory drugs Used in the control of arthritis and rheumatism, gout and inflammatory conditions of the spine.

Areas of assistance

An area of assistance is an area or system of the body that is instrumental in helping to remedy disfunctions in other parts, even though the area in question may seem to have no particular relationship to the illness. Frequently the assisted area is in the same zone. Details and examples are listed below.

Condition	**Assisted area**	**Why?**
Shoulder conditions	Hip area	Because it is in the same zone and creates a balancing effect on the structure of the body
Hip conditions	Shoulder	The same
Asthma and all allergic and respiratory conditions, including eczema	Digestive system and adrenals	Allergy usually starts in the digestive system in infancy; also the lung and digestive system are in the same five zones
Knee conditions	Lumbar spine	Most knee conditions other than specific troubles such as arthritis in the knee are caused by compression of lumbar spinal nerves
Eye and ear conditions	Kidney	It is the same zone, and medically it is known that the eyes are affected in kidney conditions
Infertility (if a hormonal imbalance)	Endocrine	Irregular cycles are often caused by hormonal imbalances
Infertility (from organic causes)	Reproductive system	Could have nothing to do with the hormonal system
Pains in calf	Lumbar spine and entire circulatory system	Could be spinal compression in the lumbar area or a circulatory problem in the legs. Is frequently a condition with diabetics

Condition	Assisted area	Why?
Weakness in hands, tingling in fingers	Cervical spine	Compression in the neck
Any under-active condition such as an under-active thyroid	Work on the adrenals to stimulate the body	
Any over-active condition	Work on the solar plexus to calm and avoid adrenals	
Vertigo (dizziness)	Often helps to work the cervical spine	Improves nerve and blood supply to the head area
Lumps and cysts in the breast	Endocrine system	Is frequently an endocrine imbalance
Palpitations (racing heart)	Often stomach area	Unless there is a known heart condition, indigestion can cause pressure from the stomach on the heart and create these symptoms
Depression	Endocrine system	Often a hormonal imbalance
Exhaustion	Thyroid/adrenals	Helps stimulate the body
Heart conditions	Liver/thoracic spine	Liver has a great responsibility in the circulatory system; controls the clotting factor. Spinal nerves in the thoracic spine help heart muscle function
Constipation	Liver/spine	Gall lubricates the bowel and the lumbar spinal nerves stimulate nerve function to the pelvic area

CHAPTER 15 The do's and don'ts of reflexology

Do not offer a cure. Professing to be able to 'cure' anything is rather a bold statement. The aim of the reflexology practitioner is to be able to relieve pain, improve bodily functions, break down stress and tension and restore the body to a far better state than it was in previously. 'Curing' really means restoring the body to a near perfect state permanently. There is no treatment anywhere, whether in the orthodox or complementary medical field, that can offer this.

Many people are relieved of their disturbing symptoms and attend for an occasional treatment – say, every six weeks – and find that this 'maintenance treatment' keeps them in tip-top condition for years and years. Many of my patients have been attending my surgery for fifteen years. Other patients prefer to have their treatment sessions, gain the maximum possible improvement in their health and then stop treatment altogether and just see how their health continues. It is not unusual for patients to return to their original practitioner after a seven-year gap. Patients always come back to where they have received the greatest benefit to their health.

Is it possible to give a course of reflexology treatments?

Generally speaking, the average person responds very well in six sessions conducted on a weekly basis. Some people take longer, and in most instances the chronic states take a little longer to improve than acute problems. The best way is to give your treatment sessions weekly until the patient remarks that their pains or symptoms have greatly improved, and at that stage to lengthen the appointment gap to fortnightly. If a good result has been maintained over a fortnightly session, then it is totally safe to see your patient in a month. After the month's gap, if all symptoms and pain levels have failed to return, it is a very good indication that a good result has been achieved with reflexology. It is then up to the patient to decide whether they wish to return once every six weeks for a general 'maintenance treatment', or cease reflexology treatments altogether and just see what happens.

Do keep all information strictly confidential

To keep good records of your patients is essential. It is also essential to make sure that information which they give to you will be in the strictest confidence. You must maintain your system of record keeping and practice management to exactly the same standards as your general practitioner would.

Don't change your techniques

There is never any need to change the practical reflexology technique which you have been trained to use with the British School of Reflexology. The technique is superb and works beautifully without any changes needing to be made. I have been using the same techniques now for twenty years, and the achievements obtained in a variety of chronic and acute medical conditions still never fail to surprise and delight me.

You do need advanced training, though, to keep you in touch with medical advances both on the complementary side as well as the orthodox side.

It is not possible to be a practitioner of reflexology, or any other science which involves treating sick people, if you know little or nothing about the causes of disease and dysfunction. It is therefore practical and sensible to attend the further training courses offered in your school where you can extend your knowledge of illness and the treatment of disease. Patients feel very safe in the hands of a practitioner who is not only proficient at their skill but is also able to communicate with patients in an informed manner on their own particular illness or disease. It gives a secure feeling to a patient when the rapport between the therapist and themselves is such that they feel confident that the reflexologist's knowledge is extensive enough for the symptoms and condition to be understood. *Knowledge instills confidence!*

How much pressure is needed for it to be effective?

Sufficient pressure should be applied to be totally acceptable to the patient without causing them any undue distress or for them to feel the need to withdraw their feet from your hands. (For the patient to do so would indicate a very bad reflexology treatment.) It does not 'take a sledgehammer to crack a nut', and as long as the pressure is consistent and applied in a professional manner which is enjoyable for the patient this is a good guide to its efficacy and the expertise needed.

I usually ask my patients, 'Is this pressure sufficient for you or am I able to go into the foot with a deeper pressure?' Obviously, it is the patient who is receiving the treatment, and you must be guided by what is acceptable to them.

You will need to use a much firmer pressure when treating (as an example) the size 11 foot of a tall man than the small foot of a child of five. This is just common sense. It is pointless working over anybody's foot with a 'feather touch technique'. This would create no benefit for the patient whatsoever. There is a need for a firm, consistent pressure with the thumb and a comfortable support for the foot at all times.

No additional aids

The greatest thing about reflexology is that we do not need any additional aids. It is a very simple form of treatment, and all we need are two hands, which will be trained to work in a precise, professional way, and knowledge, which we will gain from the professional training courses – and, obviously, a patient to whom we can apply our expertise. No oils, creams, lotions or probes or any form of electrical stimulating devices are necessary to give a good reflexology treatment. It is a 'hands-on' treatment with a total one-to-one communication between patient and therapist during the whole course of the treatment session.

Patients with infectious illnesses

It is inadvisable to treat a patient during the acute stage of an infectious illness. Reflexology is a stimulating science, and tends to create a detoxifying effect on all the eliminating functions of the body – that is, the lungs, kidneys, bowels, sinuses and skin. During an acute infection, the body is desperately trying to rid itself of an accumulation of toxins. Disease manifests itself when within 24 hours the body fails to eliminate all its waste matter efficiently. What happens is that the body stores toxins which eventually reach a very high level; disease then takes the form of your 'cold' influenza attack, eczema state, respiratory problem and so on. If we work, therefore, on those eliminating functions of the body during any acute infectious attack, we are just encouraging the body to eliminate even more toxins and this will make the patient feel even more disturbed and unwell than before.

By all means work on the pituitary gland in cases of high temperature – this has a good result in lowering temperature. Work on the relaxation techniques to create a feeling of relaxation in the patient, but do avoid those organs of elimination at the acute stage of an infectious illness. It is best to begin treating the patient after they have got over their illness, in the 'passive' state.

Patients with long-term health problems

I always suggest, when treating patients who have had a long-term history of frequent medication and perhaps are in rather poor health, that the reflexologist under-treat on the first occasion. Use a very light pressure; do not exceed half an hour of working over the feet, and just wait for a report from the patient as to how they feel the day after their treatment session. You might ask whether they feel that their condition has worsened, if they had any bowel or bladder problems, whether they were suffering from a severe headache, and so on. Be guided by these reactions. In the case of an elderly person who suffers extreme reaction to a treatment session, for example, it would be quite unlikely that they would return for a further appointment.

If all is well after the initial treatment and the patient reports a general feeling of improvement and well-being, then it is quite in order to increase the duration of the treatment session and perhaps use a slightly more intense pressure. Remember, the patient is your guide.

Can reflexology be dangerous?

There are no dangers attached to reflexology, as we are only treating a reflex point in the foot that links to a part of the body. We are not applying any undue pressure on the body, as would happen in the case of an osteopathic treatment. We are not giving the patient any medications to ingest into the system. We are not putting any creams, oils or lotions onto the feet which could perhaps affect skin tone.

The greatest benefit that we can achieve with reflexology is total relaxation and, as stress is the cause of most disease, we are well on the way to defeating a host of illnesses that people suffer by eliminating emotional stresses which affect the functions of the body.

I have treated patients suffering from heart conditions and strokes, pregnant women, brain-damaged children to name but a few, and have had some outstanding results in all aspects of health.

There are some circumstances where I would use extreme care, and they would simply be for the diabetic who has very frail skin tone on their feet with perhaps poor circulation. I would not be very happy about treating diabetics if they had any breaks in the skin area such as an ulcer on the foot or something of this nature. It would be best to wait until these problems have been healed by appropriate medical treatment.

It is quite safe to treat pregnant women. Pregnancy is a natural function and most women find that reflexology is of tremendous assistance in helping to stop fluid retention, to keep their blood pressure normal and to avoid distressing episodes of back pain. There would be just one circumstance where I would refrain from giving treatment in pregnancy, and that would be when a patient coming to me had a history of frequent miscarriage, say, at twelve to fourteen weeks. I would be much happier to wait until this period of time had elapsed as, when a miscarriage does occur, patients go through a period of grief and normally look to blame somebody for the miscarriage, and it would be very unfortunate if reflexology were to be linked to the reason for their miscarriage.

If patients suffer conditions such as verrucae, it is quite safe to give treatment providing the verrucae area is covered with a sticking plaster.

Post-operatively reflexology is very helpful, as the shock and distress associated with surgery is something which I feel reflexology is very effective in countering. Surgery also has a debilitating effect on the immune system, and again reflexology can be of benefit in restoring the immune system in the body.

Is it safe to give reflexology treatments daily?

It is totally safe to treat patients daily, although it is very unlikely that the average person will be able to attend for a daily session for practical and financial reasons. However, a member of your family or a friend will be able to enjoy a daily treatment session, and it is particularly beneficial when treating acute back conditions such as sciatica, lumbago, disc lesions, and so on. It is also of benefit to treat asthmatic sufferers every day in order to try and relax their lungs and heart function and to benefit their general health.

Can I treat the very elderly or the very young?

It is totally safe to treat everyone, regardless of age. I have treated infants under a year old and my oldest patient was 99 years old.

Do I need to get permission from a medical doctor before commencing treatment?

There is absolutely no need to get permission from the doctor or anybody else involved in the medical profession before commencing treatment with the very safe, effective methods of reflexology.

Always remember that your body is your own responsibility, it is not the doctor's, and it is really up to all of us to seek out the best form of relief and support that we possibly can. Most people have a reflexology treatment when all else has failed. They have tried their doctors, drugs and hospital treatment, and maybe have had surgery, and still their condition prevails and they find that reflexology is an acceptable treatment and one which they feel gives them maximum support.

Be realistic in your aims

If you are a practitioner of reflexology treating patients regularly, you will need to decide for yourself what are your specific aims and the relief that you expect to be able to achieve with patients suffering a variety of conditions.

It must be obvious to you that if you are treating a patient who has been confined to a wheelchair for many years suffering from multiple sclerosis, and maybe has acute and frequent bladder infections, that your talents and the relief which you would be able to offer the patient would be minimal. I expect that the main help you could offer would be to improve their general circulation and perhaps to reduce the number of bladder infections and, generally, give them a feeling of well-being thus improving their quality of life. There is no way in which a person who has been chair-bound for this length of time would be able to restore movement or walk again.

There again, if you were treating a young man who maybe had a back strain caused by the heavy physical work which he had undertaken, the achievements that you could anticipate would be total relief. Similarly, with a patient who had a long history of asthma and was now middle-aged and who for most of their life had been treated with inhalers of a steroidal nature in order for them to be able to maintain some quality of life, the results which we would expect to achieve would be a reduction in the number of attacks suffered and that these would be of less severity. It would be very doubtful whether such a patient would be able to be restored to full health and strength, as, generally speaking, long-term sufferers from asthma have quite a lot of impairment of lung function and often an enlarged heart due to the excessive strain which the heart has been under for years in coping with a very limited oxygen supply during the times of acute asthma attacks.

You must therefore take a realistic approach to the treatment of patients and understand that, although reflexology is a wonderfully beneficial treatment for a host of physical conditions, it is not the panacea to all the illnesses of mankind.

Can I treat cancer?

Many books written on reflexology warn people off the treatment for cancer sufferers. I have treated cancer patients for years, and with good results only, and although reflexology can in no way cure cancer, nor can we profess to be able to stop secondaries appearing, I have found generally speaking that patients have all exclaimed how much better they have felt. They experience a great sense of relief, and I think in the main a freedom from anxiety.

Medical doctors and researchers agree that the increase in stress and the pace of living over the last fifty years or so, plus the introduction of the western fast-food diet have made a great contribution to the increase in cancer. Surely, then, as reflexology is of admirable support in creating relaxation to the body, mind and spirit, it must be a benefit in this condition.

Many practitioners are working in hospices throughout the country. Their presence is greatly respected by the medical profession. Patients enjoy the treatment sessions and ask for a return visit and, after all, if a patient only has a very short time to live then it really is up to that patient to decide for themselves if reflexology gives them relief and a feeling of well-being.

The relatives of the terminally ill patient also find it rewarding to have been able to offer something to their suffering relative, and I think perhaps it saves any 'guilt complex' after the death of a loved one to feel that they did in fact respect any request for care which that patient asked for.

Areas of assistance

Reflexology is not just about treating the part of the body that hurts by means of the relative part of the foot. There is a great understanding of how root causes for illness are often created in another area, frequently far from the ailing part.

Pain control

It is vital that reflexologists have a good insight into the role that they are to play in the relief of pain, in the care of sick people and the benefits that are likely to be obtained with reflexology.

Generally speaking, most of the everyday conditions which one would take to the GP can be greatly relieved, and in many cases the symptoms removed altogether, by frequent treatments of reflexology by a well-qualified practitioner.

We do not diagnose, prescribe or profess to 'cure'

There has been a lot of confusion as regards 'diagnosis'. Reflexology cannot diagnose diseases within the body. However, what the practitioner can find is that a corresponding part of the foot will reveal a great sensitivity and this in turn indicates that there is congestion, inflammation and tension in that part of the body. Frequently, by treating the sensitive areas, the inflammation is relieved, tension removed and a great improvement in the functioning of the system of the body that is under duress is achieved.

When a sensitivity is found in the foot, it is absolutely wrong for the practitioner to jump to the conclusion that 'if Mrs Smith's liver reflex points reveal a great sensitivity', then surely she must be suffering from a liver disease. This is diagnosing, particularly if the reflexologist adds medical terms to the sensitivity found in the foot – 'I think perhaps this patient is suffering from hepatitis or sclerosis of the liver.'

A sensitivity in the liver can be due to many factors. It could be due to an over-indulgence in alcohol in the days before a treatment session. It could be due to an indulgence in a meal with a very heavy fat content which burdens the liver's ability to eliminate. Nevertheless, the practitioner is in no way able to diagnose these precise problems. Only doctors are able to diagnose disease; they have the facilities of X-ray machines, equipment for performing blood tests, and scanning devices and so on.

Similar situations can occur when a reflexology practitioner picks up a great sensitivity in the heart reflex area. Remember that, although the heart is a muscular area, the position of the heart reflex points within the foot also link up to the muscles within the chest (such as the pectoral muscles). These can easily become over-strained by an episode of heavy lifting, gardening or even perhaps carrying a toddler on one side for too long a period. The muscles then become over-strained, and when the foot is worked upon show up great sensitivities in the chest and heart area. It is completely wrong for any practitioner to jump to the conclusion that this person now has a 'heart condition', and it would be totally wrong and unethical for them to make such suggestions.

Reflexologists are reflexologists, and doctors are doctors, and we cannot mix the two together. There is no reason at all why, in the future, reflexologists should not work alongside the medical profession. We must always respect the many years of study that doctors have had in the treatment and care of patients, whereas the practitioner of reflexology in the main has had a very short course, which certainly does not entitle them to diagnose illness.

Aims and objectives

So, all in all, it is necessary to assess the situation which is before you and produce a realistic picture of the amount of relief you are going to be able to give your patients.

Reflexology can help in nearly all cases. In fact, we find through our long years of experience in treating people with all manner of illness that only about 6 per cent of people fail to respond to reflexology treatment. There is no real reason why these people do not get the improvement which was expected. It can often be some very simple condition which you have treated many times before but find in this instance that the patient simply does not respond. There again, there could be some very complicated long-term illness which suddenly responds dramatically to reflexology after just one or two treatment sessions. There is no real rhyme or reason why these oddities occur. Generally speaking, people who have attended treatment for at least six weekly sessions do get good results. There are very few people who attend for that sort of period of time who can honestly say at the end of the course of treatments that reflexology has done absolutely nothing for them whatsoever. However, as nothing works for everybody, we must accept that there will be that very small percentage of people who just do not respond to reflexology.

I often advise these patients to try some other form of complementary medicine, such as acupuncture, herbalism or something similar.

Conclusion

The professional support and advice offered in this book will give you, the practitioner, a guide to the development of your practice and skill as a professional reflexologist. However, reflexology can never be learnt from just purchasing a book and looking at a colourful chart. You do need the training of an expert who has been involved in the field of reflexology as a practitioner in treating patients, and as a teacher involved in the training of practitioners throughout the world.

I have shared my experiences with you. The practical application of reflexology should make it easy for you as a practitioner to work on a patient and to make the treatment session enjoyable for the patient receiving it.

Reflexology still proves to be a very safe and effective way of helping people. The only instruments we need to support our work are two well-trained hands, the professional knowledge which you will attain from our training courses and the desire and compassion to help people.

CHAPTER 16 Side effects

Side effects are the secondary and to some extent unavoidable outcome of every action or treatment undertaken. Everything we interact with has some secondary effect or spin-off, because change always occurs at multiple levels and not just superficially.

Where the intention is to improve a patient's comfort and well-being, the side effects may often be unpleasant. This chapter gives information about the risks of a wide variety of actions – from the use of medically prescribed drugs and the stress of moving house or divorce to those of eating hedgerow berries or the damage caused by acid rain and pollution. I have tried to indicate the situations where these risks are high, so that readers can decide for themselves where and how much they are at risk and can then take the most appropriate steps to limit unnecessary exposure.

When undertaking any form of complementary medicine such as reflexology, it is essential that the patient has a healthy diet, and avoids chemicals, artificial colourings and toxins.

Medical drugs

Many medical drugs are very valuable for the patient, but they are often also synthetic substances which may suppress symptoms rather than acting on the fundamental causes of the problem. Nor do they always reach the underlying deficiencies or imbalances causing the symptoms in the first place. Too often chemical remedies fail to touch the core of a problem, which may be genetic or lie deep within the personality. They may kill some of the superficial secondary bacteria but these may also include the healthy flora of the intestine. Many drugs treat only the symptoms, failing to act on the real causes, and they provoke a state of imbalance which may cause the patient chronic difficulties.

The over-the-counter sale of drugs which are freely available to you from the chemist are regarded as safe, or less dangerous than those given by prescription. Many people dose themselves for periods of weeks or months with tonics, supplements, pain-killers or aperients, believing that what they are taking is without a risk. Remember that pharmaceutical preparations are also drugs, and although their strength is sometimes less than a prescribed drug they are also potentially dangerous to your health. Even in lower dosages sensitivity reactions are common, and any medication requires caution when taken over a prolonged period.

Immunisation

Immunisation has saved many lives but it is not without some side effects. In many ways it is a natural procedure. The vaccine often contains live bacterial or viral matter which may in some cases cause a reaction. A major unresolved controversy still surrounds whooping cough vaccination. The decision to immunise an individual child should always be discussed with your doctor, particularly if you are living in a high epidemic area.

Exposure to the sun

We have all been taught to look forward to the annual two weeks in the sun and that sporting a glorious tan leads to feelings of health and vitality. Unfortunately the benefits do not always correspond to the brochures and too many are unaware of the possible risks from prolonged sunbathing and exposure to excessive heat. Some related skin cancer is increasing. The current vogue for sunbeds may not be healthy, regular use could be a factor in the development of skin cancer. High temperatures are a problem for many people on holiday and may cause an increased strain on the cardiovascular system especially for the elderly. Coaches are not always air-conditioned, and where the daily travel programme is long and tiring this can lead to illness and exhaustion.

Illicit drugs

Illicit drugs are now an issue throughout the world. Almost every town, school or college is threatened by the problem. Drug taking has become acceptable, but it is a habit which can affect young lives tragically. I have aimed to give a balanced viewpoint on the causes and prevention of drug abuse, which are extremely complex and linked to profound psychological and social problems. Often the reasons are not fully understood. The extent of the problem may reflect failure in our upbringing and educational system. Many young people no longer know how to cope with life's difficulties and wrongly believe that drugs are the short-term answer to their needs because of the myths associated with them. Drug taking is a habit that can be used as an alternative to problem solving, and when challenges occur there is a tendency to take another euphoric 'high' to gain quick relief or to evade difficulties. The more creative solution is often missed because the ways of finding it have not been taught in the past.

Approximately 70 per cent of cases seen have a stress base, but many patients are reluctant to accept some minor discomfort as an inevitable part of life, and the side effects, living in our pressurised, jet-age society. Increasingly, the patient in the surgery, like the drug addict, fails to explore their problems and the full extent of their ramifications. They are reluctant to admit their own responsibility and contribution to their difficulties.

There is a similarity between the addict who seeks a quick exit from problems through a 'fix' of cannabis and the over-anxious patient buying Codeine, aspirin or paracetamol to suppress a mild headache, or pressurising their doctor for yet another pain-killer or antibiotic.

Although most doctors resist this, patients frequently try to tell their doctors what to prescribe, often asking for strong remedies which cause side effects, when what they really need is a simple, natural approach such as staying in bed when they have flu and taking natural, restorative remedies.

The secondary effects of growing up and finding an identity and viewpoint can often be confusing and destructive to self-confidence, increasing the risk of illness. I've aimed to promote understanding of the problems and difficulties which typically occur, and once these have been acknowledged, a more positive approach and open discussion with friends or family becomes possible.

Social addictions

Social addictions are even more widespread and insidious than drug addiction and cause more deaths. For example, behind mortality from smoking and alcohol-related diseases excessive use of coffee, tea, cigarettes and alcohol reflects the needs of social props in an unhealthy society. Most people eat too much too often, so that obesity and food addiction are major health problems which affect physical well-being, psychological health and the quality of life. Dependency is now always at a high level, and in many social groups and cultures you may not be accepted if you do not drink or smoke. In a similar way you may be thought a purist or 'odd' if you don't smoke cannabis, eat meat or go to the doctor at once for a pain-killer, antibiotic or check-up when you feel unwell.

Families, peer groups and societies impose patterns of enormous pressures on children and adolescents to conform, to eat, drink and be like everyone else. Only recently expressions of individuality have become more acceptable, but it is still difficult to maintain independence in order to question authority or establish one's own ideas.

Stress

Stress is now a major threat to everyone, and an important cause of disease is now known to be a significant factor in such diverse illnesses as cancer, diabetes, heart attack, peptic ulceration, low back pain, dysmenorrhoea (painful periods), depression and phobia.

Healthy, open relationships are always important, and you should aim to keep channels of communication free and spontaneous within the family and within your treatment of patients.

Divorce is now a major stress affecting one marriage in three, and most families have at least one member who is either divorced, separated or remarried. The breakdown of a relationship always causes a great deal of anguish and suffering. Every divorce has a profound effect on any child or teenager involved, and their problems need to be handled with tact and sensitivity to avoid permanent psychological damage and reactions later in life. We all live in a gadget-conscious society, with labour-saving machinery and electronic devices in most rooms of the house. But the time saved from chores is often not used creatively. Knowing when to switch off the television, hi-fi and Walkman can avoid barriers to the appreciation of natural beauty and an awareness of reality.

Modern technology

Every gadget can be labour-saving and free you and the family from routine drudges but if used to excess they may be damaging. Television, like alcohol, is an important factor in stimulating violence, particularly in the young. It may also have far-reaching physical effects when watched for long periods too close to the screen. Other labour-saving devices such as fluorescent lighting, despite its almost universal acceptance in kitchens and offices, may cause fatigue and eye strain.

Chemicals in the home

Accidents in the home are a common family problem, with the amount of toxic chemicals stored in the garden shed and kitchen cupboard often reaching dangerous proportions. Poor or imprecise labelling creates an additional risk for the inquisitive child or handicapped member of the family. The elderly may also be at risk when depressed or confused. The side effects of accidental ingestion can be severe, and every family should educate children and the elderly members about the dangers. Never store household products near medical preparations such as gripe water, after-shave or deodorants – the labels can be confused in the middle of the night when the baby is crying or if you are tired.

Pets

Britain has more than 6 million dogs, and there are more than 10 million in the United States. Other common pets include cats, birds, rabbits, guinea pigs, mice, ponies and fish, and countless numbers of domestic animals. These can occasionally pass on diseases to humans. Although most are mild, others can lead to quite severe illness, and standards of hygiene must always be maintained when there is a pet in the house, particularly during pregnancy or if your pet falls sick. Many pet-transmitted problems are not noticed or reported, and are passed on without recognition of their origin. Problems include allergy to animal hair or feathers and other ailments such as eczema. The advantages of having a pet in the home can far out-weigh the disadvantages, but most owners should be more aware of the possible hazards.

Surgical intervention

However life saving and valuable, every surgical intervention carries some degree of risk. Many operations performed daily throughout the world have adverse physical consequences, just pain, discomfort and vomiting from the operation and the anaesthetic, though these are usually short lasting. An operation may have psychological implications for the life style and confidence of the patient, and these should be anticipated and discussed with your doctor before the operation. Hysterectomy, prostatectomy or indeed any major operation may provoke anxiety. Unless fears are dealt with openly at the time, a psychological disability may develop which is more severe than the discomfort and physical side effects of the operation.

The major emphasis in hospitals is currently on physical care, early mobilisation and rehabilitation to avoid infection circulatory and lung complications and to discharge the patient as quickly as possible. Little time is available to manage the deeper psychological anxieties which may damage self confidence.

Sexually transmitted diseases

The side effects of our permissive society include an increase in sexually transmitted diseases. The secondary unwanted effects of a sexual relationship may include AIDS, but the most common problems are non-specific urethritis (NSU), prostatis and genital herpes. Premature physical involvement or casual sex may even cause psychological problems leading to difficulties in close relationships.

The side effects of work

Occupational side effects are an everyday hazard, and to some extent every job or profession has its risks. Your office environment is important, and problems such as migraine, backache and nervous tension may be related to stress or the available equipment.

Sport and exercise

Sport is healthy and widely popular at all ages, but it can also be a strain when attempts are made to extend the limits of performance, especially in conditions of heat and humidity. Many sports and exercises, such as jogging and aerobics, commonly believed to prevent disease are not necessarily healthy for every individual, and they may even provoke problems rather than prevent them. Exercise of any kind is never recommended without consideration of the individual's age, health and vitality. Some sports carry an exceptionally high risk for the competitor, especially boxing and equestrian events. When risks are high a balanced viewpoint and personal assessment are essential.

Even yoga or meditation when used inappropriately and out of harmony with the individual can be counter-productive.

Pollution

Pollution is now a major concern for all of us, especially since Chernobyl. Leaks from nuclear plants now occur throughout the world, including Britain and the United States, and the incidence of leukaemia and cancer among those living in the vicinity of reactors has become a subject for research in many areas.

Fluoridation is a form of pollution, and though it prevents dental decay, many still have misgivings about its being an additive in our domestic water as high incidences of bone cancer, particularly in young men, have been reported in areas that have flouridation. Other environmental hazards such as radon gas, lead pesticides, nitrates, noise, acid rain and atmospheric pollution may all effect our health in a negative way.

Travel

Rapid intercontinental flight across several time zones causes profound changes in circadian rhythms, which provokes jet lag. This may be a handicap to the busy executive, the politician and also the holiday-maker, especially when delicate decisions have to be taken within a few hours of landing. The motor car too has its negative effects as well as enormous benefits, and the high number of road accidents is alarming as high-risk driving and speeding are common.

Side effects following the treatment of reflexology

We do sometimes get side effects following a treatment of reflexology. It is essential therefore that the patient and the practitioner are well aware of exactly what is going on within the body when these symptoms occur.

Reflexology is a stimulating science. It aims to improve circulation and help the body rid itself of unwanted substances. Any build-up or residue of toxins causes 'a stagnation' in one or other vital area and this in turn leads to congestion. As we apply reflexology we create a stimulating effect on the organic structures of the body which can express itself in a temporary exacerbation of symptoms.

I must make it quite clear that this in no way means that the patient has 'become worse'; in fact any reaction after treatment is something to be pleased about as it is proof indeed that the body has responded to the treatment and change is taking place. In all forms of complementary medicine – herbalism, homeopathy, acupuncture and even massage – the patient may sometimes experience a temporary worsening of their state.

The sinus area from which you are suffering may become more blocked than ever or your nose may start streaming after treatment. If you are a sufferer from migraine you may find that the treatment produces a minor migraine attack, which will be very short-term in duration but may be a temporary setback. Your back condition could feel even stiffer than before and if you suffer from colitis or any urinary tract infection you may well find that your urine output increases or you may have several bowel movements. I've even known patients to come out in a rash following the treatment session. This certainly is a very positive sign, as the body uses the skin as a first line of defence and creates an elimination area here. So any rashes or spots are in fact the body ridding itself of unwanted toxins.

One very good result following treatment with reflexology is that the patient makes a claim that they slept for many hours following a session or that night and they have never slept better in their life. This is due to a total breakdown in the stress of the body, creating within the patient a feeling of harmony and relief.

Nature needs a clean slate upon which to build her foundation of health. When we take medication for a condition we are simply embedding the problem deeper within the physical body, and from time to time we will experience another set of symptoms as the problems within the body 'burst through' and express themselves in yet another form.

It is impossible to suppress nature; she will always have her revenge in yet another part or system of the body. When treating with complementary medicines, particularly reflexology, we are treating the root causes of disease and trying to restore the balance and harmony, improve nerve and blood supply, and help the body to detoxify itself in an improved form. Once this cleansing and relaxation has occurred, then the body is in the right condition to heal itself.

There are never any dangers in treating with reflexology, and it is impossible to make a situation within the body permanently worse. As a little advice to offer as regards treating the possible side effects from reflexology I would suggest, particularly if the problems are of any organic cause, that you recommend the patient drinks a large quantity of pure spring, bottled water following the treatment session – this has the effect of flushing through the entire system and will lessen the possible side effects of the treatment. It is unusual to continue having side effects with reflexology after the first couple of treatments. Thereafter all should be plain sailing, and the patient should find that their condition improves little by little, week by week until at the end of between six and eight sessions they should have an excellent result from their particular condition.

The introduction of regular reflexology treatments gives great relief from both mental and physical stress, and patients will become aware of a new feeling of well-being which has perhaps been foreign to them until now. This is the greatest asset that this magical treatment can provide.

CHAPTER 17 Food and diet

We all have to eat to remain healthy and to replenish lost vitality from the demands of the day, but we also have a choice in what we eat, how much and how quickly. This chapter looks at the side effects of the common foods and beverages as well as the chemical additives which may also be present.

The main problems lie in imbalanced excesses and food allergy. Some people indulge in food or a diet that does not suit them because they believe it is a healthy trend or is more convenient.

There may be specific side effects from dairy products. Sugar is another possible risk and there are some less-known dangers from salt, spinach and kidney beans. In addition, there are risks in slimming aids, soya milk, cheese, and taking an excess of bran. Obesity is one of the major causes of disease in our present society. It has been linked to coronary heart disease, gall-bladder disease, cancer of the intestines and gall-bladder, accident proneness, diabetes and even a reduced life expectancy. Obesity is also associated with arthritis, varicose veins, high cholesterol and low back pain. Eat less fat and take less sugar in your diet, and exercise more, is good advice for most people.

Restraint and balance is the best advice for all ages. As much as possible, avoid excesses and food with chemical additives, and eat sensibly. Moderation is recommended in all things, and nowhere is this more true than at the table. Eat fresh produce, wholemeal bread, and raw fruit and vegetables whenever possible, and what feels right for your appetite, age and activity levels. A little of what you fancy does you good is a wise statement, but it should only be a little.

Acidity and diet

Cadmium may be released from galvanised kitchen utensils when in contact with acid foods, and it is now considered to be a major health risk. Cadmium causes birth defects and it is estimated that 250,000 babies are born each year with congenital abnormalities which are the direct result of cadmium poisoning.

Galvanised iron containers are no longer recommended in the kitchen and especially for cooking acid fruits and jam. There is a similar but less severe problem of cooking acid fruits in aluminium pans, especially apples or rhubarb. This may result in a high aluminium uptake into the body, leading to possible problems such as constipation, as well as more general toxic effects.

A high acid diet may be associated with an increased tendency to dental enamel erosion. This is especially so with a high fruit diet; also canned drinks with a low pH. Wine, if acid or young, may exacerbate arthritic problems or lead to acute gastro-intestinal problems. The worst offenders are often the acid fruits – oranges, pineapples, tomatoes, grapefruits and lemons. These are best avoided if they aggravate painful arthritis conditions or gout. They may be allowed back into the diet later when the condition has improved.

Bran

Vegetable fibre is an essential additive to every healthy diet and a major factor in preventing constipation. It should, however, be treated with sensible caution because it also has some risks when taken to excess.

Ideally, bran should be taken only as natural bran and not used supplemented with salt and colourants or sugar, when it may become a risk rather than a support to health. Bran should, if possible, always be from organic sources. If it is not, there is a slight risk that sprayed pesticides and toxic residues concentrate in the bran layers of the wheat, rye or oats and become a long-term health risk. Taken without large quantities of liquid bran can cause severe congestion in the intestines.

Diet imbalance

Food is the most important and pleasurable part of the day for most of us, but it is not always healthy, particularly if any one item is taken to excess. There are known to be risks from a high intake of dairy food because of the lipid (fat) and cholesterol content, and both have been implicated in heart disease.

Sugar is often a negative factor in such diverse problems as diabetes, hypoglycaemia, teenage acne, dental caries and obesity. Maintaining a balanced diet is important for everyone. What we eat, how food is prepared, and the way it is eaten have a profound effect on physical and psychological health.

Because health consciousness has now become a major public issue many people take vitamin and mineral supplements daily like sweets. When taken over a prolonged period of months or years with no real understanding or reason for doing so, your internal balance may be seriously undermined.

One cannot assume that anything taken routinely is necessarily healthy or right just because it is labelled as a health product. Any substance taken to excess can be harmful.

Food and exercise

Recent research shows that after regular exercise there is a fall in the circulating lipid fat levels, especially the low-density lipoprotein and higher levels of the more healthy, high-density lipoprotein (HDL).

Low-density lipoprotein cholesterol clings to the artery walls, creating blockages and leading to heart attacks. HDL helps remove cholesterol. The best prevention for heart attacks is a low-saturated-fat diet and regular exercise; at least a brisk 2-mile walk daily would stimulate the pulse rate without causing strain.

The prevention of cardio-vascular disease

Many doctors now believe that the best approach to heart problems is prevention by correcting bad eating habits in childhood. Many teenagers already have raised cholesterol levels, and good eating habits should start early to prevent adult atheroma (hardening of the arteries). Children should eat more low-fat meals, avoiding fatty foods such as chips, crisps and fried foods. They should also eat fewer biscuits and chocolate, and avoid convenience foods. It is important for every child to avoid snacks between meals, and to drink low-fat milk and lean meat where there is an existing weight problem.

All children need regular exercise, such as swimming or a sport which stimulates the heart rate and increases their health and vitality.

It is now recommended that not more than 30 per cent of all energy should be derived from fat in the diet. Children should also eat less sugar and carbohydrate-rich food and avoid rich desserts and second helpings, especially if there is a weight problem. The reduction of weight will help to keep blood pressure at optimum levels for the future. One-third of teenagers now smoke regularly by the age of sixteen. A child's lifestyle often sets the pattern for adult health, but if corrected early could help prevent many adult cardio-vascular problems at a later stage. Hereditary factors are also relevant to heart disease, as they are in some forms of cancer; for example, breast cancer. These genetic markers are now being specified for cardio-vascular disease and with advances in genetic engineering it may be possible to eradicate cardio-vascular disease in the future.

Food and cancer

Many doctors now advocate a reduction of foods which may initiate or act as triggers to cancer. Comparisons with the eating habits of people in Japan and the United States, both industrial countries, show quite opposite cancer patterns. Cancer of the breast, colon and prostate are rare in Japan, but cancer of the stomach is more common than in the United States. This form of cancer is now thought to be caused by eating smoked or salted raw fish. Families migrating from Japan to Hawaii or California have breast cancer at the same levels as the local indigenous population, as do migrants from Poland, where breast cancer is also rare.

In countries where most calories come from cereal and grains or complex carbohydrates, the mortality rate for breast cancer is much lower. Where most dietary calories come from fats, meat and vegetable oils with increased sugar consumption, the breast cancer mortality increases. The same is true of colon and prostate cancer.

In the United States, the intake of animal and vegetable fats has risen by 40 per cent, and the consumption of cancer-protective complex carbohydrates such as potatoes, and flour has fallen by 50 per cent. The US incidence of gastric cancer has fallen due to a decrease in the consumption of salted, pickled and smoked foods, which may cause nitrates to be converted into nitrites, believed to be carcinogenic. However, such formation can be largely blocked by the vitamin C content in fresh vegetables and fruit. There has also been an increase in the use of refrigeration to prevent food deterioration.

Fats which may act as preventive agents of cancer are often those rich in linoleic acid, which is found in corn, sunflower and other plant oils. Oils rich in oleic acid, present in olive oil and fish oils, do not act as cancer promoters. Eskimo women, with their oily fish diet, have low incidences of breast cancer. The same low levels also apply to Greece, Spain, Italy and other Mediterranean countries where olive oil is used for food preparation. The reasons for this are not yet known: there are suspected links between a high dietary fat intake and the prostoglandins, affecting the amount of prostoglandin synthesis. One theory suggests that oleic acid inhibits the conversion of linoleic acid to the hormone-like prostoglandins which regulate body actions, including the immune system. Prostoglandins may also act on mid-brain hormone centres which control breast tissue development and the release of the breast hormone prolactin.

The cruciferous vegetables, such as cauliflower, brussels sprouts, broccoli and cabbage, contain indoles and isothiocynates which are currently thought to block tumour activity and to be cancer-protecting agents.

Other significant trigger factors in cancer may be a lack of cereal fibre or a diet low in vitamins A and C. Low levels of selenium may be another factor in cancer formation.

Foods high in saturated fats

Diets high in saturated fats are thought to be associated with cardio-vascular atheroma (hardening of the arteries). Such diets are also linked to high body cholesterol levels and heart attacks, and also to obesity. The main sources of saturated fats are dairy products, meat, especially red meat, also avocados, coconut oil and palm oil.

Men from Finland and the United States may have high coronary rates because of their high dietary fat intake. There is, however, a lower incidence of heart disease in Japan, Corfu, Crete and Dalmatia, where fat intake is lower.

At present, the average American takes 40 per cent of their calories from fats. Many doctors believe that this should be reduced by half, to 20 per cent, and the amounts of raw foods, cereals, fibres and fruits, increased for health.

An article in *Scientific American*, in November 1987, stated that prehistoric man consumed only 10 per cent of his total dietary calories as fat, with a high ratio of unsaturated to saturated fat and a daily fibre intake of at least three times the present average (15 grams). (The intake of prehistoric man's vitamin C was also estimated at four times that of the average US citizen in the 1980s.)

Modern diets have changed appreciably since the beginning of the Industrial Revolution about 250 years ago. Fat levels have risen as food became a status symbol. At the same time fibre intake has been reduced, and refined sugar has been introduced into the diet at high levels, which have increased steadily.

Flatulence

Flatulence, or gassy abdominal distension, is mainly caused by odourless gases such as nitrogen, carbon dioxide, methane and oxygen. Odour is caused by skatoles and indoles, hydrogen sulphide, volatile amines and the presence of short-chain fatty acids. Swallowing air can lead to increased amounts of nitrogen in the intestinal area.

Some artificial sugars are believed to be an important factor causing flatus. The major sugars concerned are sucrose, raffinose and stachyose, which are not well digested and pass into the colon, where the action of normal intestinal flora (organisms) causes the formation of carbon dioxide. Fermentation within the large intestine of the indigestible fibrous part of beans, peas and soya products may also cause gases to be formed. Onions also cause gas to be formed.

Flatulence can be considerably reduced by taking charcoal as a biscuit or as activated charcoal to reduce gas formation. Fermentation of soya-bean milk with lactic cultures (yoghurt) also helps. For most people, the best cure is an avoidance of any food which does not agree with them and which tends to form excessive wind and gases in the large intestine.

Food additives

There are reported to be approximately 3,500 different food additives in use, equivalent to 200,000 tons every year. The amount increases by 5 per cent each year, with a near-average intake of 8lbs of chemicals per person per year. In the last thirty years the amount of food additives has been estimated to have increased tenfold.

Where instant convenience foods are regularly used, the amounts will be far higher. Of the 3,500 foods, only about 350 have specific legal controls, and fewer still have been fully tested. About forty food additives are widely suspected of being cancer-linked. E150 caramels have been associated with cancer; also the preservatives E245-252 are suspected of being carcinogenic because they are nitrates, which react with foods or bacteria in the body to form nitrites which may be a cause of cancer. They are also thought to reduce the ability of blood to transport oxygen. Other food additives are believed to cause allergic reactions and hypersensitivity in adults as well as children. They include colourants, flavours, emulsifiers, texturisers, gelling agents, anti-oxidants, thickeners, preservatives, meat colourants and tenderisers.

All colourants and dyes should be used with care; they have been withdrawn in Norway and are heavily restricted in Sweden. For health reasons, only choose food for its smell, taste and freshness, and not because of its bright colour. Tartrazine (E102) is an orange-yellow dye additive, which is widely used to give food more appeal and to make it more eye-catching. It is a synthetic coal-tar derivative, chemically related to benzoic acid. Tartrazine is often present in fizzy drinks, orange squash, multi-coloured sweets, canned vegetables, chewing gum, frankfurters, macaroni, spaghetti, bread, butter, cheese, concentrated fruit juices, ice-cream mixtures, jellies, pickles, relishes, sherbert, toothpaste, lozenges and on the surface colouring of many medicines. Between 20 and 40 per cent of people who are sensitive to aspirin are also believed to be sensitive to tartrazine. When there is a member of the family with aspirin sensitivity, it may be wise to avoid all tartrazine-coloured foods and also pills where it is used in the capsule or coating.

For many years tartrazine has been widely considered to be a major trigger factor for hyperactive, restless behaviour in children or teenagers, causing hyperkinesis, often with irritability and disturbed behavioural problems. Modern research has not been able to confirm the hyperactivity theory. Tartrazine has also been suspected of being a trigger to attacks of skin sensitivity, rashes from foods – particularly urticaria, dermatitis and asthma, hay fever and possibly bladder irritations, bladder weakness and bed wetting. Tartrazine in adults has also been linked to hot flushes, general malaise, weakness, palpitations, blurred vision and depression. Other tests have shown a relationship with nasal congestion, sneezing, hoarseness, sweating and drowsiness. If you are treating any patient with an allergic reactive background – such as asthma, hay fever, skin rashes, eczema and the like – it is of immense importance for them to learn to avoid all colourants, particularly tartrazine, in order to get the best effect from your reflexology treatment sessions.

Diet and the elderly

It is important for elderly people to have a balanced diet as well as regular exercise such as walking or swimming. Often the taste for sweet foods does not change as we get older; it may even increase to unhealthy levels with the desire to eat cakes or biscuits and sugar at the expense of more nutritional items, especially foods with vitamins and protein. Many elderly people do not experience thirst, and consequently may not drink enough. The diet should be kept varied and interesting. Elderly people should eat little and often, the main meal being at lunchtime rather than in the evening. Where budgets are low, inexpensive sources of protein are milk (preferably low-fat milk), eggs and fish, but lentils and legumes (peas and beans) are also good protein sources. If necessary, these can be purchased in tins as they do not lose their protein if preserved in this way. However, the elderly should also aim to eat as much fresh food as possible for a balanced food intake.

A lentil dish and a glass of milk with a piece of cheese or a portion of yoghurt is the protein equivalent of a piece of meat. Salt intake should always be kept low because of the risks of causing a rise in blood pressure and developing cardio-vascular problems. Elderly people should avoid alcohol or only take it in moderation.

CHAPTER 18 Don't blame it on the weather

The poor old British weather gets the blame for most of our aches and pains, sniffles and sneezes. We proclaim that if we sit in a draught or go out in the wind or get exposed to low temperatures then we are going to catch colds or flu. There again we still grumble when it is hot, because we then say that germs and viruses absolutely thrive in the heat causing 'summer colds', gastro-intestinal infections and the like.

Generally speaking, the weather is not the cause of illness. The cause of disease is when the body fails to eliminate from the liver, the kidneys, the lungs, the intestine and the skin all its toxic elements. In such circumstances, we have an overloaded system; viruses and bacteria thrive in this destructive element. It was Louis Pasteur who proclaimed, 'Don't worry about the viruses, worry about the soil in which they grow'. So, if the soil is right, disease flourishes.

It is very common to hear of some epidemic early in the New Year and then it is always blamed on the grey, dark, dismal days of January, cold temperatures, high winds and the damp environment. Although looking out on to this type of 'grey day' is not very stimulating to the mind and certainly does not make us feel at our best, it is still not the main cause of illness. More than likely the main cause of an infectious spread of anything is simply because after Christmas and into the New Year we have done an enormous amount of indulging in very high calorie, fat- and carbohydrate-based foods, our alcohol intake has probably been higher than at any other time of the year and consequently our bodies are totally clogged and congested and are having a struggle to eliminate all their waste efficiently. So we find that the virus or bacteria which attacks us and gives us a bout of flu, gastric flu or a heavy cold is simply the result of over-indulgence through the Christmas period.

The air around us and the rain are good for the body, they are good for the skin, and fresh air never did anything but revitalise and improve our circulatory and respiratory function. Why, then, do we, the British, always look for the cause of illness in an external environment? Disease is created from within, never from without. Apart from the exceptional circumstances when people in underdeveloped countries are living on inadequate supplies of food and in areas where there is open sewerage so that dysentery and cholera are rife, our health should be unaffected by weather conditions. You may find that when you have some epidemic in your office it is not every single member of staff who goes down with the illness. Although the viruses must be multiplying in their billions in the warm surroundings of an office where numbers of people are working together in the same space, it does not necessarily follow that the illness will affect everyone. There could be one member of the staff who, whatever happens, does not go down with Asian flu or something similar, and that is because that person's body is in a far less congested state than other people's.

Disease also manifests when we are in a very low mental state, when our interest in life has declined, when we feel we have no real function or purpose or direction, maybe when we are suffering from a very painful, recent loss of a member of our family. Our immune system will be greatly affected by negative emotional feelings of this kind, and it is normal that when a person is under a lot of stress they will find that their health deteriorates, that they fall prey to almost any illness around.

I am sure you have heard it said, 'I seem to catch everything that's going around'. All that antibiotics and drugs do is simply to suppress the symptoms. Remember, you still have the underlying cause, the congested body, so therefore, until you resolve this, you are very likely to have a recurrence within a week or two. It is quite common if you take an antibiotic for a respiratory infection – sometimes if the infection is severe and seriously affects breathing then we do have to resort to these measures – to find that a couple of weeks later you have an episode of diarrhoea and sickness. This is the body's way of trying to get rid of the congestion which is still there.

A purpose to life

I remember a very moving story told to me at a meeting I attended recently, quoted from a book, *Man's search for a meaning* by Victor Frankel. Victor was one of the prisoners in the death camps in Germany during the last war. Within a few months of being taken to the camp he saw the atrocities that occurred within, and despite his weak, painfully thin body, he decided that he was going to try to survive because he wanted to be able to write about the experiences he saw, so that never again could these terrible things happen to man. So you see, Victor had a real purpose for living. Confined in his cell, Victor wrote about the experiences he witnessed. Had any of the notes which he wrote been discovered of course he would have been instantly put to death, but somehow he managed to hide his papers and keep this very vital information. One day he was taken with a hundred other prisoners into the dreaded gas chamber and he felt sure that this was the end. To his and the other prisoners' amazement when the jets were switched on above them they found that it was not gas, it was ice cold water that came out of them. These prisoners, naked men, were standing under these ice-cold jets in sub-zero temperatures for hours. Remember that they were all in a terrible state of emaciation, were just mere skin and bone, some had a lot of sores and scarring to the body from mutilation and torture, but as Frankel said in his book, the joy of experiencing this ice-cold water rather than choking gas was more than he would ever have expected, because here there was hope. He was not going to die on this particular day, he had a purpose and was still alive. During the hours of exposure when icicles formed and hung on the naked bodies of all the prisoners, icicles attached themselves to the nose, the fingers and any extremities that they could get a hold on and then the water was turned off.

Many of the prisoners had frozen together. Nevertheless, they were returned to their cells and not one single person from those hundred prisoners ever contracted pneumonia, a cold or flu or anything else. The reason was that they were so determined to survive and they were so exhilarated by receiving cold water rather than toxic gases into their bodies that the life force was stimulated at their chance, at the very smallest chance, of survival.

Over the next weeks most of the prisoners who went through that torturous episode were gassed. However, Victor was one who did survive, and he survived and lived to write the book from which I am quoting this story, and despite the most terrible ill health, the torture, the damage to his body and the emaciation, he did survive and he survived because he had real purpose and direction – a search for meaning.

How then can it possibly be that we who are living in such a comfortable environment, as most of us do today, with heating, lighting, plenty of food, fresh air (although I must confess it has become more polluted of latter years), and most of us have some sort of income, even if sparse, how can we then blame all our aches and pains on to the weather? If you look at this chapter again you will perhaps have a better understanding of how it is the mind that has the greatest influence on whether or not you survive ordeals that may come your way.

The importance of the family

People who are loved, wanted and supported and are within a close partnership have far more chance of survival from any traumatic episode in their life than solitary individuals who perhaps have lost all their main family and are living in a lone state. Every developmental stage of life poses some degree of physical and psychological challenge. The most dependent stage of life is infancy, but to some extent dependency is present throughout life. Babies are physically vulnerable and their major problems include wind and colic, diarrhoea, infection and dehydration, also obesity and failure to thrive. Many psychological problems originate from a variety of causes at this time. A healthy infant may become ill very suddenly but also recover just as quickly. Psychological damage is less dramatic at this stage but can also occur, especially when a child is neglected, made anxious, abused or is unwanted. Although every baby can make loud demands for its physical needs, it may be less able to express psychological needs for recognition, affection and closeness.

Children sense if their parents are ill or stressed, and this can have an effect on the sensitive child. The parents also need to be aware of the emotional needs of their child as well as physical ones, particularly as these are usually expressed by non-verbal means. The same needs are intensified in adolescence and may cause problems in establishing mature relationships and being self-confident if not dealt with sensitively, particularly where there have been major traumas in early childhood.

In adults with a close relationship, physical and emotional dependency needs are usually fulfilled through the intimacy and closeness of the couple, but should the relationship break down early infantile patterns may reassert themselves in the forms of eating, smoking or drinking to excess and neglect of a balanced diet. Indigestion, colic, flatulence and peptic ulcers are some of the common physical symptoms experienced by adults under stress, particularly during a divorce. Feelings of rage, depression, anger, confusion and apprehension, with demands for instant solutions, may also resurface at this time. The monthly hormonal cycles affect women both physically and emotionally, and the 24-hour circadian (biological) rhythms affect mood, drive and energy in both sexes.

Pregnancy

Pregnancy is a period of life which gives fulfilment and satisfaction but is also a time of major physical adjustment to accommodate the foetus and the birth process. These changes exert a great deal of pressure on the mother, who must also at the same time relate and respond to the needs of other members of the family as well as her own. Fathers go through psychological changes at this time too, sometimes identifying with the mother. They may develop physical symptoms associated with the pregnancy or birth, including nausea resembling morning sickness and abdominal swelling, mimicking a phantom pregnancy.

In the community most emphasis is put on the physical needs of the mother for care during the ante-natal and post-natal periods, but mothers also experience periods of emotional pressure at this time which are not always sufficiently recognised or acknowledged. These include doubts, fears, feelings of isolation or inadequacy which can lead to depression and, in severe cases, to a nervous breakdown or mental illness. The physical and psychological duality continues into middle age, and whenever there is strain or problems are not fully declared and worked through they may be expressed in a preoccupation with dieting, weight loss, sometimes gambling or agoraphobia or an attempt to find comfort from problems by over-indulging in food. The underlying needs are still present, however, for closeness, understanding and to be acknowledged, and until these are dealt with the physical manifestations may not respond to treatment.

The menopause

The menopause usually affects women from about 40 onwards. It is a period of physical and emotional adjustment. The classic symptoms of apprehension, sweating and palpitations are most marked in women. Hormonal and psychological changes and adjustments also occur in men at this age.

The elderly

Problems occur in the elderly because they become physically and emotionally stiff and rigid. When the early experiences of feeling closeness are positive, problems which occur in later life, such as adapting to change, a new home or environment, are also easier to resolve. Like the child, the elderly person is vulnerable to heat, cold and fluctuations in temperature. Many of the common circulatory disorders which occur at this time are either associated with a diminished body surface area or impaired temperature regulatory mechanism.

The elderly also have emotional needs, and when these are not fully or instantly met, like the child they can also react with extremes: with panic, agitation and emotion. Delusional ideas occur when these anxieties and fears become exaggerated, although they are often quickly resolved by reassurance.

Whenever an adult becomes intolerant of change or fixed in their ways this can create problems. With the elderly, often a change in the psychological or physical environment can become a threat and lead to infantile behaviour or panic, although at other times and in the same environment they are perfectly well and healthy, often very positive and creative well into old age.

CHAPTER 19 Reference guide to treating specific conditions

Condition	Symptoms	Main area to treat
Addison's disease	Adrenal insufficiency causing wasting. Hypertension. Vomiting	Whole of endocrine system
Alzheimer's disease	Degeneration of cerebral cortex. Loss of memory and paralysis	Extensive work on whole of spine and brain, preferably daily
Ankylosing spondylitis	Disease of joints, destruction of joint space followed by sclerosis and calcification, resulting in rigidity of spinal column and thorax	Spine, brain, shoulder, hip, knee, coccyx and pelvis. Adrenals to help break down inflammation
Arteritis	Inflammation of arteries	Heart/lung, thoracic spine, adrenals
Bronchitis and asthma	Inflammation of bronchial tubes. Spasm of the bronchioles, resulting in difficulty in exhalation	Heart/lung, adrenals, thoracic spine (to help nerve supply to thoracic area), digestive system (often a weakness in the digestive system causes excessive mucus in the system)
Bursitis	Inflammation of a bursa of a joint	Work the relative joint; i.e. knee/elbow etc., plus lumbar spine in the case of knee (cervical spine for elbow). Helps the affected nerve supply to part

Condition	Symptoms	Main area to treat
Candida	A fungus that causes thrush	The whole of the intestinal and reproductive area
Carcinoma	Cancer of the epithelial tissue	The whole of the body, especially spleen to help the immune system
Carpal tunnel syndrome	Numbness and tingling in the fingers and hand as the result of compression of the median nerve of the wrist	Cervical spine and elbow area to aid nerve supply to wrist
Cataract	Opacity of lens of eye	Eye, sinuses, cervical spine
Cerebral haemorrhage (stroke)	Rupture of an artery of the brain due to either high blood pressure or disease of artery	Entire spine, brain, respiratory, circulatory and kidney (to help renal blood supply which would ultimately help blood pressure)
Cerebral palsy (spasticity)	Condition in which the control of the motor system is affected due to a lesion resulting from a birth defect or deprivation of oxygen at birth	The spine and brain (work this area frequently during a treatment 6 or 7 times up and down each foot)
Cervical spondylosis	Degenerative changes in the intervertebral discs in the cervical spine	The entire spine and chronic neck area
Chole-cystitis	Inflammation of the gall bladder	Liver and gall bladder area
Colitis, diverticulitis and irritable bowel syndrome	Inflammation of the colon	Entire digestive system and lumbar spine to help nerve and blood supply to the pelvic area
Conjunctivitis (eye condition)	Inflammation of the conjunctiva	Eye/cervical spine and all sinus areas
Constipation	Difficulty in passing a motion	Entire intestine and liver/ gall bladder (bile helps lubrication of the bowel) and lumbar spinal nerves

Condition	Symptoms	Main area to treat
Crohn's disease	Chronic form of enteritis affecting terminal part of the ileum	Entire intestine
Cystitis	Inflammation of the urinary system, mainly affecting the bladder	Urinary system. Coccyx, pelvis and lumbar spine
Depression	A feeling of gloom	Entire endocrine system to help balance hormonal output. Lots of work on relaxation techniques
Diabetes	Caused by a deficiency of insulin production of the pancreas	Digestive, endocrine, circulatory and respiratory systems
Dysmenorrhoea	Painful or difficult menstruation	Work urinary and reproductive and coccyx/ pelvis and lumbar spine
Eczema and all skin diseases	Inflammation of the skin	Treat as for asthma (comes from the same source)
Emphysema	The over-distension of the lungs by air. Distension of the alveoli of the lungs due to atrophy of the alveolar walls	Treat as for asthma
Endometriosis	Inflammation of the endometrium (uterus)	Reproductive and endocrine, can be a hormone imbalance
Epilepsy	Disorder of brain marked by the occurrence of convulsive fits	Brain, spine
Fibroid	A tumour composed of mixed muscular and fibrous tissue in the uterus	Reproductive system
Glandular fever	Infectious illness of the glandular system	Endocrine, respiratory and circulatory system
Haemorrhoids	Varicose veins in rectum	Intestinal area, in particular descending colon and rectum

Condition	Symptoms	Main area to treat
Hay fever	Allergic rhinitis	Sinus, ear, eye, adrenal
Headache	Pain in head	Entire spine, brain
Hepatitis	Inflammation of liver	Liver, digestive system and adrenals
Hypertension	High blood pressure	Circulatory and respiratory and kidney. **Do not** work on the adrenals when treating high blood pressure
Hypotension	Low blood pressure	As above, **but work** on adrenals to increase levels
Incontinence	Absence of voluntary control of the passing of urine or faeces	Urinary/intestinal, lumbar spine, coccyx, pelvis
Indigestion (dyspepsia)	Failure of the digestive process	Digestive and intestinal areas
Insomnia	Inability to sleep	Spine, brain, respiratory and circulatory systems
Lumbago	Painful condition of the lumbar muscles due to inflammation. May be caused by displaced intervertebral disc	Coccyx, pelvis, lumbar spine
Mastitis	Inflammation of the breast	Breast, shoulder, endocrine system
Mastoiditis	Inflammation of the mastoid bone in the ear	Head, neck, ear, cervical spine
Meniere's disease	Giddiness resulting from disease of the internal ear	Head, sinuses, ear, cervical spine, chronic neck
Migraine	Paroxysmal attacks of headache usually with nausea, also preceded by disorders of vision	Head, neck, spine, liver (migraine is often digestive in origin and the liver is usually affected)
Multiple sclerosis	Degeneration of the myelin sheath covering central nervous system	Spine, brain
Myocarditis	Inflammation of the myocardium	Respiratory, circulatory and thoracic spine

Condition	Symptoms	Main area to treat
Nephritis	Inflammationn of kidney	Urinary system, lumbar spine
Neuralgia	Pain in the nerves of face	Facial area, cervical spine, all sinuses
Oedema	Abnormal amount of fluid in the tissues causing swelling, particularly in ankles	Urinary system, circulatory and lumbar spine and lymphatic area surrounding groin
Orchitis	Inflammation of testicles	Reproductive, coccyx, pelvis, lumbar spine
Osteoarthritis	Disorder due to excessive wear and tear to joint surfaces, affecting mainly weight-bearing joints	Work out thoroughly the prime joint or part of the body affected, and spine and urinary system to encourage good elimination
Pancreatitis	Inflammation of pancreas	Digestive system
Phlebitis	Inflammation of veins	Circulatory and respiratory systems
Prostatitis	Prostate inflammation	Urinary and reproductive, also lumbar spine
Retinitis	Inflammation of retina	Eye, sinuses, chronic neck
Rhinitis or hay fever	Inflammation of nose	Sinuses, nose/throat, digestive system (often a food allergy), adrenals to reduce inflammation
Salpingitis	Inflammation of fallopian tubes	Entire reproductive, endocrine systems, plus coccyx. Pelvic/hip
Sciatica	Neuralgia of the sciatic nerve	Lumbar spine, coccyx, pelvic/hip, sciatic area
Sinusitis	Inflammation of an air sinus	Sinuses, eye/ear, cervical spine, facial area

Condition	Symptoms	Main area to treat
Spondylitis (as in ankylosing spondylitis)	Inflammation of a vertebra. Condition of unknown origin occurring characteristically in young men. Ossification of spinal ligaments with ankylosis of the cervical and sacro-iliac joints	Entire skeletal system
Tennis elbow	Inflammation of bursa of joint, affecting the insertion of the entensor tendon of the forearm muscles	Cervical spine, shoulder, elbow
Thrombosis	Coagulation of blood in the vessels	Respiratory, circulatory systems, spine
Thyrotoxicosis	Hyperthyroidism. Excess of production of thyroxine	Thyroid and all endocrine glands
Tinnitus	Ringing in the ears	Neck, ear, sinuses
Tonsillitis	Inflammation of the tonsils	Throat, sinuses, cervical spine (thymus gland) (in young children to help immunity)
Trigeminal neuralgia	Pains in the face of unknown cause	Face, sinuses, eye/ear, neck
Vertigo	Giddiness	Ear, sinuses, cervical spine

CHAPTER 20 The treatment session

It is important to place your patient in as comfortable a position as possible. Therefore, the use of a treatment couch or one of the portable footstools, known as a 'portaped', should be available. The 'portaped' is ideal in as much as it can be adapted for use, i.e. lowered and raised to fit at the end of an armchair, garden lounger or similar. It is very light and so is ideal for any home visits.

Do not use oils or creams, an oily foot makes it very difficult to isolate the reflex points. A very light dusting of baby powder is all that is needed.

The recommended order of treatment

Begin with the right foot and use the *side to side relaxation exercise* (see Figure 3.1). Repeat the same procedure on the left foot.

Return to the right foot and use the *diaphragm relaxation exercise* (see Figure 3.2). Repeat the same procedure on the left foot.

The *diaphragm relaxation exercise* gives a great feeling of relaxation to the patient, in as much as it slows down the respiratory rate, creating a sense of peace, very similar to the experience you have when you are 'just dropping off to sleep'.

The right foot

We are now going to concentrate our work on the right foot.

Order of Treatment	Figure references
1 Work up the plantar side of the lung. (Remember to work from medial to lateral then lateral to medial.)	5.4 and 5.5
2 Work down the dorsal side of the lung/breast area.	5.6 and 5.7
3 Use the *metatarsal kneading relaxation exercise*.	3.3
4 Work up all the toe areas. (You will be working out both the endocrine area in the brain as well as the sinuses.)	10.7 and 10.8

	Order of Treatment	Figure references
5	Work out the eye and ear area.	10.9 and 10.10
6	Work out the neck/thyroid (plantar side first then the dorsal).	8.4 and 8.6
7	Work out the coccyx, pelvis and hip.	11.3 and 11.4
8	Work up the spine over the brain, the chronic neck and front of the face. (Working out the skeletal system simultaneously works the central nervous system.)	11.5, 11.6, 11.8, also 10.14
9	Work down the spine.	11.7
10	Work out the shoulder area.	11.9 and 11.10
11	Work out the knee/elbow area.	11.11
12	Work out the primary sciatic area.	11.12
13	Work out the secondary sciatic area.	11.13
14	Work out the liver area.	4.9 and 4.10
15	Use the 'hooking out' technique on the ileo-caecal valve.	4.13
16	Work out the entire intestinal area to the base of the heel (this includes the buttock and back of the hip area).	4.14 and 4.15
17	*Ankle freeing relaxation exercise.*	3.4
18	Work out the bladder, ureter tube to kidney.	12.4
19	*Under and overgrip relaxation exercise.*	3.5 and 3.6
20	Work out the area of the uterus/prostate ovary/testes/fallopian tube/ vas deferens.	13.5, 13.6, 13.7 and 13.8
21	*Foot moulding relaxation exercise.*	3.7
22	*Rib cage relaxation exercise.*	3.8

Record at this stage the sensitivities found on the right foot on your Patient's Treatment Record Card.

The left foot

You have already worked on the left foot with the side to side relaxation and diaphragm relaxation exercise when you began treatment, so there is no need to work over that area again.

	Order of Treatment	Figure references
1	Work up the plantar side of the lung.	5.4 and 5.5
2	Work down the dorsal side of the lung/breast area.	5.5, 5.6 and 5.7
3	Work out the heart area.	6.4
4	Use the *metatarsal kneading relaxation exercise.*	3.3
5	Work up all the toe areas.	10.7 and 10.8
6	Work on the eye and ear reflex.	10.9 and 10.10
7	Work on the neck/thyroid (plantar side first, dorsal side second).	8.4, 8.5 and 8.6
8	Work on the coccyx, then pelvis and hip.	11.3 and 11.4
9	Work up the spine over the brain, the chronic neck area and front of the face.	11.5, 11.6, 11.8, also 10.14
10	Work down the spine.	11.7
11	Work out the shoulder area.	11.9 and 11.10
12	Work out the knee/elbow area.	11.11
13	Work out the primary sciatic area.	11.12
14	Work out the secondary sciatic area.	11.13
15	Work out the stomach, pancreas and spleen.	4.11 and 4.12
16	Work out the transverse descending and sigmoid colon to the base of the heel (this includes the buttock and back of the hip area).	4.16, 4.17 and 4.18

Order of Treatment		Figure references
17	*Ankle freeing relaxation exercise.*	3.4
18	Work out the bladder, ureter tube to kidney.	12.4
19	*Under and overgrip relaxation exercise.*	3.5 and 3.6
20	Work out the area of the uterus/prostate ovary/testes/fallopian tube/ vas deferens.	13.5, 13.6, 13.7 and 13.8
21	*Foot moulding relaxation exercise.*	3.7
22	*Rib cage relaxation exercise.*	3.8

Record at this stage the sensitivities found on the left foot.

Return to the right foot and just work over the sensitivities on the right foot two or three times.

Repeat the same procedure on the left foot.

You should find that the sensitivities have already decreased which means that you have effected a good treatment session.

You should aim to complete your treatment within an hour.